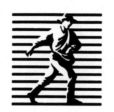

ALSO BY
DANIEL CALLAHAN

ABORTION:
LAW, CHOICE AND MORALITY

THE TYRANNY OF SURVIVAL

SETTING LIMITS

Medical Goals in an Aging Society

Daniel Callahan

SIMON AND SCHUSTER

NEW YORK · LONDON · TORONTO · SYDNEY · TOKYO

COPYRIGHT © 1987 BY DANIEL CALLAHAN
ALL RIGHTS RESERVED
INCLUDING THE RIGHT OF REPRODUCTION
IN WHOLE OR IN PART IN ANY FORM
PUBLISHED BY SIMON AND SCHUSTER
A DIVISION OF SIMON & SCHUSTER, INC.
SIMON & SCHUSTER BUILDING
ROCKEFELLER CENTER
1230 AVENUE OF THE AMERICAS
NEW YORK, NY 10020
SIMON AND SCHUSTER AND COLOPHON ARE REGISTERED TRADEMARKS
OF SIMON & SCHUSTER, INC.

DESIGNED BY EVE METZ
MANUFACTURED IN THE UNITED STATES OF AMERICA

10   9   8   7   6   5   4   3

LIBRARY OF CONGRESS CATALOGING IN PUBLICATION DATA

CALLAHAN, DANIEL, DATE
  SETTING LIMITS.

  BIBLIOGRAPHY: P.
  INCLUDES INDEX.
  1. AGED—UNITED STATES—SOCIAL CONDITIONS. 2. AGED—
UNITED STATES—ECONOMIC CONDITIONS. 3. AGED—MEDICAL
CARE—UNITED STATES. 4. AGED—GOVERNMENT POLICY—
UNITED STATES. I. TITLE.
HV1461.C35 1987   362.1'0880565   87-13029
ISBN 0-671-22477-8

FOR
ELLEN McAVOY
AND
ROSALIE MILLER
AND IN MEMORY OF
ROBERT S. MORISON

Contents

Preface

A QUESTION I WAS FREQUENTLY ASKED while writing this book was whether, in my old age, I would be willing to live with my own recommendations. Would I be prepared to have life-extending treatment stopped? Would I decline an organ transplant that might give me in my old age a few more good years? I do not know how I might react. Some people hang on to life, others let it go, and I do not know which kind I will be. I can only now say that the writing of this book has forced me to think intensively about the course of my life and what aging will mean to me, what it is already coming to mean for me. I wrote this book between the ages of 56 and 57, and I know that statistically speaking, I have a good chance of living to 80 or beyond. My mother lived to be 86, though my father died at 62. To which of them will I be closer in the age of my own dying?

I was told that a few people, shocked at what they had heard of my thesis, speculated that I might be going through a late mid-life crisis. They may have been right, but not for the right reasons. To paraphrase the old joke, there is nothing like spending months thinking about old age and death to focus the mind. If it was not the result of a mid-life crisis, it surely provoked one. I looked at my children with a new eye, trying to think about what happens to people over the span of a lifetime. I looked at the old with a new eye as well, trying to understand where they now stood in their own eyes, in their own lives. And I tried to look at myself in some fresh way, poised as I am on the edge of old age, whose tracings I can already discern. Would I be willing to live with my own recommendations? The question came back to me time and again as I thought about the problems.

This much I can say. There is little danger that the views I advance here will elicit such instant acclaim (or any acclaim, for that matter) that the present generation of the elderly will feel much of their effect. That could take two or three decades if there is any merit in what I say, and what I am looking for is not any quick change but the beginning of a long-term discussion, one that will perhaps lead people to change their thinking, and most important, their expectations, about old age and death. That kind of timetable would mean that my age group would probably be the first to feel its impact, not those who are now old. It is my generation, and those who are still younger, for whom this book is most pertinent. I will be much better able to live with my own recommendations if, over the coming years, we all begin to change the way we think about aging and death. My own expectations will have changed, as will those of the people who care for me.

I have, in any case, presented my ideas because some significant change in our thinking about health care for the elderly is needed. I do not think we have any other realistic choice but to ask, once again, some basic questions. Our present course neither will nor should work. This book is an attempt to devise an alternative approach. I hope I would have the nerve to live with it.

The writing of this book had the advantage of some most helpful arguments, discussions, and manuscript readers. Although they did not see the final manuscript, Bernice Neugarten, Malcolm Morrison, Elaine Brody, and David Thomasma provided important initial help in commenting on my original outline. They were, for the most part, sharp critics of what I proposed to say and forced me to alter my original plan. While they may still not be happy with what I say, I hope they will see that their help made a real difference. Harry R. Moody, Nicholas Rango, and Thomas Cole were careful and astute readers of an early draft of the book. In Moody, Rango, and Coles

I encountered a group of scholars who were bringing some new and bracing perspectives to studies of aging. Norman Daniels shared with me the manuscript of his own new book on aging and commented perceptively on my manuscript. He has pioneered the way on these issues. In Sissela Bok, in particular, I had the help of a longtime friend and someone who has thought long and deeply about our understanding of aging. Dan Brock read a later draft of the book and called attention to many flaws and unresolved problems in my argument.

My colleagues at the Hastings Center, particularly Susan Wolf, Willard Gaylin, and Bruce Jennings, were unstinting in their help, as was Lauri Posner. My Hastings Center assistant Paul Homer was, at 25, the youngest reader of my manuscript, and his grandmother, Mrs. August Homer, was, at 80, the oldest. This book, I should note, represents my own views and not those of the Hastings Center.

I have dedicated the book to three people who have meant a great deal to me in recent years. Ellen McAvoy has been my much-admired administrative assistant at the Hastings Center for fourteen years and an indispensable organizer of my life. Rosalie Miller has managed the Center's finances and has brought both care and dedication to her work. The other person to whom this book is dedicated is the late Robert S. Morison, a former professor of science and society at Cornell and MIT, who had read and astutely commented on the first draft of this book and had received the second when he died at the age of 80. He was a man who spent much of his life thinking about the meaning of life and especially of old age and death. To me and to many others he was the very model of a wise person. He manifested just those traits I commend in this book: an acceptance of aging and death together with a mind that was lively, probing, and engaged until the very end. I am sorry that he will not see how much of this book bears the mark of his influence on me.

Although they had nothing directly to do with this book, my friends Eric Cassell and Leon Kass have much to do with some of its central themes—those of the ends of medicine and the relief of suffering. For many, the name of Kass in particular will evoke the recollection of the debate generated by former Governor Richard Lamm of Colorado when he spoke out in 1985 on terminal care for the aged. His remarks were interpreted—mistakenly, I believe—as advocating that the old get out of the way to make room for the young. He also cited some writings of Leon Kass about the biological value of aging and death. Since I cite some of those passages also in this book, and know and respect both Kass and Lamm, some might conclude that this book was stimulated by that earlier debate. It was not, though it is fair to say that we have all been worried about the same problem, that of setting limits in a technological society and determining what are sensible and proper human ends. My own history with this issue goes back to the first years of the Hastings Center, in the early 1970s, when Robert S. Morison, Eric Cassell, Leon Kass, Hans Jonas, Paul Ramsey, and a number of others first tried to understand the meaning of death and its significance for medical practice. I am forever thankful for the seriousness, imagination, and care they brought to those troubling, difficult issues.

I thank, finally, my wife, Sidney. She encouraged me to write this book, and then had to live with it for many months, as one idea after another was tried out on her, and one draft after another given to her for still another reading. It was a rich, if also troubling, time: aging and death are not light matters. Their existence is, however, the best possible evidence of how much we need each other. They should not be faced alone.

Daniel Callahan

1 | Health Care for the Elderly: How Much Is Enough?

NOT FAR FROM WHERE I LIVED as a child was a restaurant of a kind once known as a "tearoom," a respectable but modest establishment catering heavily to older patrons. Among them were a number of women whose circumstances I had trouble understanding. They were elderly and often frail, but most mysterious was their solitude. Once in a while two elderly women would be eating together, but most often each was alone, dining delicately and slowly, obviously drawing out as long as possible the ritual of nourishment and life in a public place.

I was touched and disturbed. Why were there lonely old women like that? It seemed wrong—not the way lives should draw to a close, and not what I had come to expect. The elderly women I had known, my grandmothers mainly, had been surrounded by family, at the center of a circle of respect and deference. That was one image of old age, as power and authority. My mother presented still another. Not for her their somber dresses, their restrained laces at the neck, their utter disregard for makeup. She was the forerunner of a new kind of old person, someone who had a large circle of friends, who fought to stay young, whose clothes were always bright and gay, and whose hair was dyed blond into her mid-8os. At the restaurant I saw still another possibility: that of old age as isolation and loneliness. Only later was I to visit a nursing home and to learn even more, about old age as a time of crushing physical and emotional burdens for some, and life as a trouble to be endured until the release of death.

My parents said nothing about any of this to me, though I can recall my mother some years later talking about how difficult it had been for her to take care of her elderly mother, that same mother who seemed to me (rightly enough) so powerful in her sway. Then as now, it was the women I remembered; the men either died earlier or, if they lived, faded to inconsequentiality. I cannot say that as a child I made any coherent sense of these conflicting images of old age, nor was it at the time a situation that anyone seemed to worry very much about. Old age was taken to be inexorable, and whether it turned out for good or ill was mainly a matter of luck. Yet I was left with a puzzle, one that has become all the more acute as the years have passed. How ought we to understand old age: as a time of new prospects and horizons, or of imposing wisdom and power, or of decline and inconsequence—or some bewildering mix of all these possibilities?

As it turned out, much has happened to the aging between my childhood, in the 1930s, and the 1980s. The dramatic changes began to take place during the 1950s and 1960s, and flowered fully by the 1970s. A decade or so ago there was a combination of great indignation and great optimism. The indignation was directed against "ageism," that debased stereotyping of the elderly as poor, useless, and senile. Not true, any number of newly formed interest and advocacy groups were saying. The optimism was based on some solid new trends. Poverty among the aged was dropping. Many elderly were beginning to discover exciting new social roles and opportunities. The traditional idea of inevitable physical illness and senility overlooked the powers of the new biomedicine to cure the old no less than the young. The average life expectancy continued to increase, and even more striking gains in life extension were possible. The dawn of a new era of medicine intertwined with a new era of aging seemed to be at hand.

The process by which the transformation of old age became a goal of medicine in recent decades was part of a larger story. The historical development of biomedicine has meant two things of profound importance: the gaining of immense new knowledge and technical powers, and a transformation in our understanding of life and its possibilities. These developments can be understood as three different stages, each building upon and eventually reinforcing the last. The first stage brought changing ideas of medicine; the second generated different notions about the nature of health; and the third is now producing different ways of thinking about what we can hope for from life and about the way a life can be lived.

1• Changing the Conception of Medicine. The greatest transformation of medicine over its long history has come only within the past century: a decisive movement from primarily caring to caring and curing. For most of its history, medicine was relatively powerless to do much about illness, disease, and death. It could offer only comfort and palliation: humane care, not efficacious cure. That situation began to change by the middle of the eighteenth century, primarily because of better diets and sanitation. By the nineteenth century, the scientific method was coming to be applied to illness and disease. Systematic biomedical research first appeared. By the early twentieth century, medicine began to offer real cures; no less important, it became scientifically ambitious and managed to convey that ambition to the general public.

By the end of World War II, the cumulative impact of the scientific approach—from immunizations through antibiotics to high-technology diagnostic and curative devices and methods—began to show in increased life expectancies and reduced rates of crippling illnesses. After the war, an all-out scientific attack on disease was mounted. That attack included major budgetary allocations to biological research, the declaring of "war" against cancer, heart disease, stroke, and any number of other afflictions. At the same time, the provision of health care was coming to be understood differently. With the 1965 Medicare and Medicaid programs, a public commitment was made to adequate health care for the elderly and the poor. While caring would still receive strong support—and would remain a basic aspect of actual practice—curing, not caring, became the triumphant ideology. First by its commitment to a scientific methodology, and then by its harnessing of the power of the state for research money and a comprehensive delivery system, medicine had simultaneously changed its self-conception, its place in society, and public expectations about its social contributions. Contemporary medicine is an arena for constant high-technology innovation, a massive and profitable industry, and an inescapable element in national economic prospects and welfare. The needs of the elderly, themselves redefined by the medical advances, offer the richest possible terrain for medicine to exercise its powers and its aspirations.

2• *Changing the Conception of Health.* The great transformation in the nature of medicine could not, however, have come about without a corresponding shift in the concept of health. What do we want from biological understanding, applied medical research, and access to health care? We certainly want to be free of crippling and fatal disease, have an intact body, and be helped to overcome our various accidents and infirmities. We want, put simply, "good health," that universal desire of those of all ages, but particularly of the elderly, who far better than the young understand its value. But what are we to count as good health, or a decent life span, or bodily wholeness? Those are increasingly hard questions to answer, primarily because medical progress constantly pushes forward the frontiers of health. It invites, indeed seduces, us to set an ever-higher standard of what should count as "good health" and an acceptable life span. It exhorts us to reject fatalism and a passive acceptance of the limitations and natural decay of the body. The message from medicine about our health is clear enough: it is no longer luck or chance that some live and some die but, instead, simply a failure of science yet to succeed in managing or conquering those illnesses which remain. They are *all* open to systematic biomedical attack. There is no reason to suppose that they will not be as amenable to cure or control as, say, the whole range of infectious diseases—typhus, smallpox, diphtheria, and the like—which are now only distant memories in developed societies.

The power of this picture, of ever-improving good health as a realistic goal, has had a number of consequences. It has stimulated the development of a notion of health that encompasses mental as well as physical well-being, and (in the 1947 World Health Organization definition of health, for example) the hope and belief that happiness, not simply bodily welfare, can be encompassed as well. The support of biomedical research and access to health care have as a consequence taken on the high status of basic human rights and entitlements. How could it be otherwise when medicine can so decisively save and improve life? What can be had ought to be had. Where better to work out the full implications of that principle than in the lives of the elderly, where health can become so fragile and death is always so near?

Not only has health been transformed as a medical goal and social ideal, but the place of good health in individual lives and the body politic has been no less transformed. It has moved from the sphere of the accidental and fortuitous—where death was once the companion of all age groups, beyond the help of medicine, politics, and economics—to the realms of high science and established psychological and political expectation. The technological imperatives that transformed the nature of medicine from caring to curing have no less profoundly affected our idea of health, moving it from a nebulous hope to a fundamental human and social requirement. What can be done medically ought to be done. What ought to be done ought to be available to all. What ought to be available to all becomes the moral responsibility of all. In that set of propositions the elderly have seen their medical hopes and needs enfranchised.

3• Changing the Conception of Life. It is but a short step from a changed conception of health to a changed conception of what it means to live a life. Effective contraception and safe abortions, for example, mean that women can now effectively think of themselves in roles other than the maternal. An extended life span means thinking about the stages in life, and the possibilities of life, in new ways. Not only are the facts of life changed, but also the meanings associated with them. At the minimum, as we now know, the period between the coming to maturity of one's children and the end of one's life can be significant, not years but decades. That shift of course casts childbearing and child rearing in a different light. It becomes a temporal phase, no longer a temporal centrality. It has the same unsettling but exciting effect on conceptions of work, leisure, and retirement. The old landmarks of the stages in life no longer apply, or at least require radical revision to continue making sense.

The changes effected by biomedical advances appear to have at least three important consequences for the understanding of what it means to live a life. They profoundly alter, first of all, our perception of our capacity to control our life, strengthening a belief that our medical destiny lies in our own hands—individually by virtue of better personal health care and sensible precautions, and collectively by a commitment to basic biomedical research and improved health-care delivery. There is, second, an alteration in the way the consequences of our actions are understood. By breaking what seemed to earlier generations fixed cause–effect relationships, actions once hazardous can now yield tolerable outcomes. The obvious example of the biological sundering of sexual activity and procreation is more than matched by the increasingly effective sundering of illness and old age, no less open to scientific intervention.

A third consequence has been to encourage the belief that the long-standing, seemingly inherent finitude of the body—and, through drugs, of the mind and emotions—can be overcome. Only the most scientifically euphoric will talk of a total conquest of aging and illness. But it has become routine casually to entertain the idea of doing away with cancer, heart disease, and stroke (the great remaining killers of the elderly), and with arthritis and dementia (which can make old age such a misery). To the extent that our sense of life's possibilities must contend with the constraints of illness, the threat of a premature death, and the untoward health consequences of our actions, to that extent will a change in the way we think about health result in a deep change in the way we think about life. Whether we *are* our bodies or merely inhabit them is one of the oldest of philosophical questions. Yet there is little doubt that when we begin to transform the way we think about our bodies, we are well on the way to transforming the way we think about our lives and about our selves. Correspondingly, an expansionary vision of health, because of its proved value to change life, will continue to shape our understanding of medicine and its possibilities. Medicine becomes not just a way of curing or controlling disease, but no less a way of trying to cure or control the problems of life.

Aging has forever been one of those problems—acceptable for some but fearsome for most. Yet we have come a long way in bringing old age to heel. We now expect to live relatively long and healthy lives. We think we have a right to such a life, or that it is at least a normal and perfectly reasonable expectation. A premature death offends the new and improved longevity odds, and thus the way things ought to be. Society, most people believe, has an obligation to help us achieve that good health which has become our natural birthright, through its investment in medical research and its medical entitlement programs. Yet good health and a long life are still not quite enough. What good are they if old age cannot be a time of satisfaction, continued personal fulfillment, and social respect? In asking questions of that kind, we have also come near to claiming that old age is a time when we have a right to an optimistic outlook, when old age is (true enough) the last stage of life, but a potentially long one that ought to afford its own distinctive benefits and attractions.

Yet if medicine has brought a new way of thinking about life's possibilities, there have also been some shadows. If most of the elderly are better off than in earlier generations, poverty and isolation continue to afflict elderly women and minority groups to a grossly disproportionate extent. Medicare by no means covers all medical expenses of the elderly, and out-of-pocket costs can bring some old people close to destitution. Should they require nursing-home care, as some 5 percent will each year, they must achieve destitution as a qualification for Medicaid support. Far from profiting from old age, many elderly people seem to have their lives preserved too long, well beyond the point of continuing satisfaction and meaning. The "death with dignity" movement has tried to cope with this, but while achieving some success, it has failed to overcome the technological imperative of contemporary medicine to extend life. Longevity has brought still other problems. The specter of Alzheimer's disease, so far both terrifying and incurable, has added some new fears to old age. If many of those who have been called the "young-old" (65–75) do better than their predecessors, those over 75 (the "old-old"), and even more those over 85 (the "very old") may do very badly indeed. The success of acute-care medicine, which can save lives in ways unimaginable even a decade ago, has generated a sharp increase in chronic illness. Lives are saved, but lives that will be sick until death finally wins out. The great killers of the elderly—heart disease, cancer, and stroke—have yet to be cured; and with increasing longevity, not only do they (except for heart disease) occur more often, but so do other wasting diseases as well.

| Old Age as Social Avalanche?

YET NONE OF THOSE PROBLEMS is necessarily intractable, and with time many of them could be ameliorated. But there is a set of developments that is new, posing some inherently more difficult dilemmas. Is it possible that medicine's triumphant reconstruction of old age has also unwittingly created a demographic, economic, and medical avalanche, one that could ultimately (and perhaps already) do great harm—a demographic avalanche by harmfully increasing the number and proportion of the elderly and also, in the process, distorting the ratio of old to young; an economic avalanche by radically increasing the burden of social and familial dependency; and a medical avalanche by lengthening life beyond a capacity to preserve its quality? It is, and should be, uncomfortable to even raise a possibility of that kind, especially when there is so much yet to be done. Old age is still no idyll, even for those in good shape. Many aged are in desperate straits; medicine still has considerable good work to do. We are, moreover, only now perhaps beginning to appreciate the possibilities of old age for opening up new human frontiers. Even in a time, then, when rapid social change is daily fare, the idea that the humane medical care and cure for the elderly sought in the 1960s and 1970s could turn out to be the occasion of a new social threat in the late 1980s and 1990s is hard to accept. Yet it seems to be true, however appalling and distasteful the idea may be.

The general trends in the number and proportion of the elderly, and their health-care costs, are striking, and though I have put more details about those trends in an appendix (page 225) it is well to keep a general sense of them in mind. Between 1900 and the present, there has been an eightfold increase in the number of those over the age of 65, and almost a tripling of their proportion of the population. Those over the age of 85—the fastest-growing age group in the country—are 21 times as numerous as in 1900. In 1985, for the first time in American history, the number of those over the age of 65 came to exceed those under the age of 18. In the early 1960s, less than 15 percent of the federal budget went to those over the age of 65. By 1985, that percentage had grown to 28 percent. A little over $80 billion of private and government money was spent on health care for the old in 1981; that is expected to grow to $200 billion by the year 2000—and in constant 1980 dollars. Public expenditures are expected to rise to $114 billion.

Given figures of that kind, it is not unexpected perhaps that uneasiness has begun to appear about expenditures on the elderly. Three complaints in particular have been heard. The first is that an increasingly large share of health care is going to the elderly in comparison with benefits for children. Is that fair and sensible, and how far should it be allowed to go? The second is that a disproportionately large portion of health-care expenditures goes for the care of the elderly dying. Is that a wise way to spend our money, and is it actually greatly beneficial to the elderly? The third is that a large and growing proportion of health-care research and technology is devoted to conditions that affect the elderly more than other age groups. Is this a creative, prudent, and just way of using the possibilities of biomedical research?

These complaints might seem to bear only on the allocation of resources, at best a matter of making good use of increasingly limited funds; and that is part of the story. I see them as symptomatic of even deeper, more disturbing problems: of the way we understand aging and death, of the relationship between individual and common good, of the proper goals and ends of medicine and biomedical research, and of the moral bond between past, present, and future generations. While I will touch upon the economic and other social issues of what has come to be called "intergenerational equity," it is those latter issues I am most concerned to explore.

I will make many references to the "old," the "aged," and the "elderly," and will use those terms interchangeably. What will I mean by them? For the most part, I will simply mean those over the age of 65. There is now great pressure to push back the time when old age is said to make its onset, to 70 or even 75. My own observation is that 65—though arbitrary in many obvious respects—is not nearly so bad an age for policy and other purposes as it is often made out to be. That an increasingly large number of people, the majority, are in good health and vigorous at that age, and that many can and should continue to work, need not preclude what I think true, that the beginning of old age is by then putting in its appearance in almost everyone. When, however, I am referring to those well along in their aging, or those who are very old, I will try to say so.

The plan of this book is as follows. Chapter 2 opens the discussion by focusing on the question of how we should now, in the light of medical progress, understand aging. What are appropriate goals for aging and old age? In Chapter 3, I shift the focus to the ends of medicine. Given the potentiality of an unending medical struggle against aging and death, the new frontier of medicine, is there an alternative, more suitable goal? In these two chapters together I hope to show that we need to think in terms of the deepest ends and goals of medicine—what ought to be its point and purpose?—and that when we do so, the goals of aging and those of medicine should be analyzed together. Medicine now gives us a new understanding of the possibilities of old age; contemporary old age, in turn, gives us a new understanding of the possibilities of medicine.

In Chapter 4, I begin working out the practical implications of the viewpoint just developed. In that chapter, I examine the obligations that the young have toward the old, both in the sphere of the family, where "filial obligation" is important, and in the civic realm, where the issue of societal support of health care for the elderly is crucial. How, I ask, should family and society relate to each other in the care of the aged? In asking what is the obligation of the young to the old,

I mean to raise a question parallel to one raised in Chapters 1 and 2: whether we can speak of the obligations of the old to the young. In Chapter 5 I take on the problem of the allocation of health resources to the elderly. What is a fair way to make such allocations, particularly in light of obligations to other generations and to other social goods? Chapter 6 examines the difficult problem of terminating treatment of the elderly, those who are dying and those who may not be. Chapter 7, finally, looks briefly at the question of "intergenerational obligation," the care of the aged and the welfare state, and some parallels between prolife (right-to-life) and aging-advocacy groups on matters of health care for the aged.

I have three purposes. The first and most fundamental is to stimulate a public discussion of the future of health care for the aged. The second is to propose a different way of understanding the problems of providing that care than is commonly considered: that of using age as a specific criterion for the allocation and limitation of health care. My third purpose is actually an extension of the second: that of working through some of the details and implications of the approach I propose. There is considerable prematurity in working through some of those details, but it seems important to make the effort in order to explore the practical and other problems that would be posed if my argument is, in a general way, plausible. What would it mean in practice to have a health policy for the aged of the kind I propose? Inevitably, for all the concreteness of my specifications, that part of the book (especially Chapters 5 and 6) should be read in the tentative vein in which it was written. It should be taken seriously, but not literally. Even within the framework I propose, there is much room for argument about the details.

What matters most to me is that, as a community of the old and the young, we begin to think about where we want to go in the long run in our use of medicine to address the decline and death that have been the ineradicable marks of human aging. We have so far simply tried to use medicine to vanquish them or to keep them at bay as long as possible. That direction is no longer tenable. It is incoherent at its core and increasingly unworkable socially and economically. My approach will not be a generally pleasing one. It puts to one side the kind of relentless optimism that has been the mainstay of medical advancement and its economic underpinning. It rejects the conceit that we can have anything we want if we put our minds to it and are willing to pay for it. That has surely been the spirit of recent medical and social initiatives on old age. This book, by contrast, is a call for limits, for sobriety of purpose, and for a willingness to ask once again how we might creatively and honorably accept aging and death when we become old, not always struggle to overcome them. We may continue for a few more years to put off this kind of reckoning, to ignore these questions. Muddling through often works well enough for a time. But we have done that long enough, and if the strategy I propose is not exactly an attractive one, it may be the only plausible and fair one.

2 | Reconstructing the Ends of Aging

IN ITS LONG-STANDING AMBITION to forestall death, medicine has in the care of the aged reached its last frontier. It is not that death is elsewhere absent—for children and young adults obviously still die of maladies that are open to potential cure—but that the largest number of deaths occurs among those over the age of 65, and the highest proportion of all in those over 85. If death is to be humbled, that is where the great and essentially endless work remains to be done.[1] Yet however tempting that challenge, medicine should now restrain its ambitions at that frontier. It should give up its relentless drive to extend the life of the aged, turning its attention instead to the relief of their suffering and an improvement in their physical and mental quality of life.

So great is the desire for life and the fear of death that I have no hope such a view of the goals of medicine in the face of aging could have any persuasiveness were it to stand alone. A fresh understanding of the ends and meaning of aging, encompassing two conditions, should complement it. The first condition is that we need, both young and old, to understand that it is possible to live out a meaningful old age that is limited in time, one that does not require a compulsive effort to turn to medicine for more life to make it bearable. The second condition is that as a culture we need a supportive social context for aging and death, one that cherishes and respects the elderly while at the same time recognizing that their primary orientation should be to the young and the generations to come, not to the welfare of their own group. For the old to make an unlimited claim upon medical resources, to want the frontier of death constantly pushed back, will be seen by young and old for what it is, a danger. The old will know it represents a failure of their own highest vocation and an unconscionable demand upon societal resources that could be better deployed. The young will know that to harbor such desires for themselves when they become aged will be a poor preparation for their own old age. That will help them neither as individuals who must make sense of the full course of their own lives nor as the conservators, in their turn, of the assets needed by their own children's generation.

| The Modernization of Aging

HUMAN AGING PROVIDES an attractive target for modernization. Aging is nowhere wholly welcomed. Its ultimate effects upon the body and often the mind are destructive, and its outcome is death. If modernism arises from the aggressive desire to "do something about" the deficiencies and deprivations of that which life in the raw thrusts upon us, the process of aging is an ideal candidate. Modernism might be characterized as the belief that human ingenuity can bring about a better future, that science and unprejudiced rationality are the key instruments of that ingenuity, that nature is not fixed or normative in its ends but is malleable to human purposes and construction, and that the traditions of the past must be transcended in the light of more current insights. By the "modernization of aging" I mean, more specifically, the belief that the physical process of aging should be aggressively resisted, and that the life of the aged ought to be transformed from one of old-fashioned disengagement and preparation for death to a continuingly active involvement in life and a persistent struggle against decay and demise. Since I by no means want to hold that all the items on the modernization agenda are wrong, only many of them, it is necessary for me to proceed carefully. The question is: where should we draw appropriate lines?

A common classical view of old age was that it should be accepted and that old age was actually superior to youth because of its ripeness, wisdom, and experience. A more recent belief has been that because of the rapid pace of social change, the future is best left in the hands of the energetic and adaptable young. The modernization of aging represents a still more advanced stage: to be old is potentially (if not quite yet) better than to be young because it is the new frontier of medical progress, of personal freedom and individualism, and of styles of life that could transform industrial societies.[2] Under this dispensation, the aged are not at all a surplus group, or merely "senior citizens" serving out their time until death. They are the new pioneers. The kind of healthy, self-directing, self-realizing, past-transcending life they are now in principle able to live becomes the medical, social, and political goal, the ultimate reward of a progressive and medically enlightened society.

Can we pay for this kind of progress? Of course we can. The high costs of health care for the elderly are simply the acceptable price to be paid for creating a society whose aim is no longer only the welfare of the young, but the preservation of those now enabled to break from the biological, cultural, and familial constraints of the past. In the words of Gerald Gruman, one of the most eloquent proponents of that view: "A life span that is truly modern in attaining humanist, meliorist, and individualist values still is ahead. At present, the worth of the individual is not so much a fact as a goal. This interpretation requires confronting the truism in contemporary culture that resources should be invested preferentially in the young, because they have a future and the elderly do not. However in the furthering of a genuinely modern culture, it is the aging who actually have pride of place; they are where the action is, for they are something *new* as a large population sector. The solving of their problems is a make-or-break task for the modern forces that brought them ino being. Moreover, the elderly, as individuals, face challenges *new* to themselves which call for successive, creative renewals of identity. And as part of humanity, they live in a historically early, or *new* phase of accelerated modernization. *Thus, the aging population does have a future, as it becomes re-engaged at the frontier of modern cultural adaptation and realization through historical time.*"[3]

The wonderfully optimistic flavor of that passage articulates (even if it overstates) a perspective implicit in much current biomedical work on aging and in much of the aging-advocacy work of those who speak on behalf of the affluent, healthy elderly. The terms "modern maturity" or "prime time" have, after all, come to connote a life of travel, new ventures in education, the ever-accessible tennis court or golf course, and delightfully periodic but gratefully brief visits from well-behaved grandchildren. That this idealized picture leaves out the elderly poor, the chronically ill, minorities, and single or widowed women is beside the point. Its importance as a utopian reference point lies in its projection of an old age to which more and more believe they can aspire and which its proponents think an affluent country can afford if it so chooses. That it requires a bio-medicine which is single-minded in its aggressiveness against the infirmities of old age is of a piece with its hopes. Just as the old do not have to live, as they did in the past, in graying self-effacement, so neither do they have to tolerate the disease-riddled bodies that were the fate of previous generations. Why not in effect declare aging a disease and lavish upon it the same attention once devoted to high infant-mortality rates and smallpox? The success of campaigns against the latter provides ample ground for hope that the same can be done with aging. Why not? Why not indeed?

I confess to a certain sheepishness in judging that this wonderful idea of a modernized aging is fatally flawed. It surely and undeniably has its attractions, and I will benefit from many of them. But quite apart from some still-to-be-conquered social and biomedical realities which may prove permanently elusive—the vast increase in chronic illness that has been a part of the life extension of the elderly, the persistent and so far intractable poverty or near-poverty of a significant proportion of the elderly, the growing number of small, often fragmented families and thus most likely isolated elderly people in the future—there are more serious reasons to be skeptical. It is a projection which lacks that most important of all ingredients for old age: a sense of collective meaning and purpose. It is instead simply a prospectus for an individualistic old age as more of the same—more freedom and less responsibility, more years and less poor health—but with no illumination whatsoever about the meaning or significance of those years, no purpose or goal for which those goods are to serve as means.

But death will come soon enough anyway in this new world, even if later than in the past. There is nothing in that modernizing aspiration which promises to respond to the present root problem of aging, that of the need for a respected place for old age in society and in the lives of individuals. It may actually create new problems, at once offering no real alternative for the aged but to follow the crowd in their struggle against old age while at the same time draining resources from other societal needs.

Before turning to the question of how old age is to be given fresh meaning, I want to linger on some of the details of the modernization project. I single out those offered by Gruman because his are the most fully sketched and part of a rounded, plausible approach to aging. Moreover, one does not have to scratch far below the surface of much writing on aging, and particularly writings against ageism, to see how well he has managed to articulate a good part of its animating impulse. He presents in a vivid way what is usually obscured.

At the heart of Gruman's version is a mixture of two cultural traditions: that of the Italian Renaissance humanism of Luigi Cornaro, with is emphasis on a long old age marked by wisdom, hedonistic pleasure, and amelioration of the harshness of nature; and that of the Enlightenment (especially Condorcet's) with its goal of improving life generally while also specifically lengthening the life span and staving off death. Death is not to be passively accepted any more than a disengagement by the elderly from the world should be accepted. Just as death and the tradition of "medical mortalism" (that death is the inescapable defining limit of the physician's activity) ought to be rejected, so also should a division of labor that allocates work functions according to age. Personal sacrifice by the elderly as a way of finding meaning in life and uniting the community, Gruman holds, should no less be rejected; creativity and self-assertion are more valuable character traits. The common view that old age represents a discontinuity in creativity is particularly objectionable. Personality and selfhood can be shaped anew at every stage of life, in old age as much as in youth. Such a creative self must, however, be one rooted in individualism and in a rejection of collectivist notions of human worth, flowering, and decline.

The aged are for Gruman not only to be comforted. They are also to be freed. The novelist George Eliot's term "meliorism" catches, finally, an ethic of action oriented toward the relief, not the acceptance, of pain and suffering. Human betterment is ever possible, and neither nature nor history is fixed. "The principal source of the prestige that modern biomedicine enjoys is the fact that it was the one professional group that seriously took up the imperative of melioristic progress from the Enlightenment . . . for biomedicine carries forward the transcendent Judeo-Christian quest for salvation from evil and death."[4]

Gruman paints a beguiling picture, and many of its features are perfectly sensible: that pleasure should be a part of old age, that the possibility of further developing the personality and self is viable, that work and its place in society can and should be reconceived to make a greater and more significant place for the elderly, and that the future is open to improvement and progress. The struggle of the Enlightenment against fatalism, against a too-ready acceptance of suffering, is a valuable part of its legacy, however unbridled that has become at times.

But Gruman's individualistic vision is deeply flawed. There can be no community at all, much less community among the generations, without some sacrifice of an unlimited quest for individualistic pleasure on the part of the old. Why should the young respect, much less help and support, old people who mean to live for their own pleasure? And since the young can understand the delights of pleasure also, why should they not—well tutored by their elders—adopt a similar value? Would that not carry with it an untoward implication, however: that the old and their claims on pleasure and the resources necessary for its full pursuit could interfere with the young's pursuit of *their* pleasure? Might not the young then conclude that they should take priority?

As for death, if there is no stance toward it in the modernizing view other than its outright rejection, then any kind of preparation for it, and acceptance of it, becomes nothing more than fatalism. This fatalism will be all the more painful because death, when it comes, will be individually and socially pointless and medically adventitious. There can be no mature understanding of life unless death is accepted as a "defining absolute" (to use Gruman's term of rejection).[5] We do not any longer have the luxury, as individuals or society, to leave what Gruman agrees are "central questions of meaning and value" endlessly "open for future resolution." That is his (and a common) way of ackowledging and then evading them. There is no reason to believe, unless we change course, that they will be resolved or even faced in the future. The goal of modernizing old age is nothing less, ultimately, than its banishment. It begins by banishing the hard question about the meaning and value and significance of old age. We need to look in a different direction.

| Old Age: Meaning and Significance

WHAT KIND OF SENSE can be made of old age, of the fact that our bodies change and decline, sicken and decay, and then die? Even if we distinguish between growing old and becoming ill, between becoming old and becoming stale, between chronological and biological age, or between our externally assigned social role and our internal sense of place—even if, that is, we make all of the distinctions recommended in the professional literature on aging, in the end death happens, and we exist no more. While old age and death are obviously distinguishable, death comes at the end of old age. How should we prepare for that moment, and what should we think about it? That is an uncomfortable question, one that most people, I suspect, would call a private rather than a public issue. It has been banished to the closed confines of church or synagogue and, if accompanied by distressing symptoms (anxiety, fear, obsession, depression), thought suitable for therapeutic and especially pharmacological intervention.

Those evasions will no longer do. The interior meaning and contours of old age ought to be public issues, no less than debates about the indexing of social security payments or of adequate housing. If the aged are to understand themselves, and if our society is to make sense of them in their increased numbers and growing demand on resources, then the meaning and significance of old age must be a matter of open discussion and of an effort to shape some social agreement. This becomes all the more important as we open a debate on the allocation of health and other benefits to the elderly. In the absence of a public philosophy on the meaning of aging, any effort to limit or reduce resources for the elderly will, with some justice, be looked upon with suspicion—as a way of appearing to say, with behavior which belies words, that the old are simply not worth any further investment. That is a possibility, but it is just as likely that the blind, literally aim-less modernizing of old age will deny it any social value. If the elderly lack an established, coherent, and meaningful place in life and society, there is no real rationale for their protection; it merely exists as a kind of sentimental benefi- cence. That is little defense against the weapon of cost containment and the reproach of budget deficits.We lack, in the end, any pen- etrating social vision of the place of the aged.

The individualism of our society is a major obstacle in the way of developing that kind of vision. It is more comfortable with worry- ing about improving the lot of individuals than coping with in- tergenerational responsibilities. It is more at home in struggling to maintain freedom of and financial support for medical research on aging than in asking how that freedom ought wisely to be used. Yet the place of the elderly in a good society is an inherently communal, not individual, question. It goes unexplored in a culture that does not easily speak the language of community and mutual responsi- bility. The demands of our interest-group political life constitute another obstacle. Such a political life places a high premium on a single-minded pursuit of the interests of particular groups or causes, is adept at using the language of individual rights as part of its campaigns, and can rarely afford the luxury of publicly recognizing the competing needs of other groups.[6] The greatest obstacle, how- ever, may be our almost complete inability to find a meaningful place in public discourse for suffering and decline in life. They are rec- ognized only as enemies to be fought: with science, with social programs, and with a supreme optimism that with sufficient energy and imagination, they can be overcome. We have created a way of life that can only leave serious questions of limits, finitude, the proper ends of human life, of evil and suffering, in the realm of the private or of religion. They are treated as incorrigibly subjective or merely pietistic.

To give old age a deep and substantive meaning, we require a strong sense of continuity with the future as well as with history and earlier generations. We need, as a people, a common conviction that old age has meaning and significance. We must have a lively tradition of civic discourse that allows difficult, highly personal matters of meaning to be openly discussed. These will not be easy goals to achieve; our culture works against them. Yet now more than ever, we do have a need for meaning, and thus a strong stimulus to search for it; and at least some of the ingredients are at hand. Before trying to outline what the latter might be, what do I mean when I speak of "meaning" and "significance"? By meaning I refer to the interior perception, backed up by some specifiable traditions, beliefs, concepts or ideas, that one's life is purposive and coherent in its way of relating the inner self and the outer world—and that even in the face of aging and death, it is a life which makes sense to oneself; that is, one can give a plausible, relatively satisfying account of oneself to oneself in aging and death. By significance I refer to the social attribution of value to old age, that it has a sturdy and cherished place in the structure of society and politics, and provides a coherence among the generations that is understood to be important if not indispensable.

An understanding of meaning and significance in old age need not be full and perfect. No reflective person is ever likely to feel that he or she adequately understands the meaning of life and death. They will remain ever-troubling matters for future just as they have been for past generations. And no society in the near future, faced with the great and constantly shifting changes in health and longevity wrought by medicine, is likely to feel utterly comfortable about the exact social significance to be assigned the elderly. The important point, however, is not the achievement of certainty. It is instead that the questions of meaning and significance are understood to be rich and worth our searching for together as a community, not merely in our private reveries or uneasiness; and that there is no obvious reason to despair that, however hard, progress can be made with them. Nor is there any reason to fear (to invoke another common fantasy) that an attempt to talk publicly about the ends of aging in a pluralistic society and what might constitute a common good of aging will lead eventually to an "official," and thus dogmatic, repressive view. It is a lack of talk which is more likely to produce that outcome.

A useful place to begin the search might be with the now-repudiated "disengagement" theory. That familiar theory, first advanced in the late 1950s just as a fresh concern for the aging was gathering speed, was meant to explain the supposed withdrawal of the aged from active social engagement and, at the same time, to explain a disengagement of society from the aged. The attributed purpose of this dual disengagement was, from the side of the individual, to allow a preparation for death; and from the side of society, to permit the old to step aside in order that the young might fill their social roles. The process of disengagement was also supposed to exhibit a reduction in the number and intensity of social roles for the elderly and, with that reduction, a reorientation of their emotional content toward the emotive and expressive. While the timing and details of the disengagement would vary from person to person and culture to culture, it was said to be a universal feature of aging.[7]

Disengagement theory was immediately and zestfully criticized and, for over two decades now, has been repeatedly assaulted by gerontologists as one of the worst of the many "myths" about aging. That the old might want to pull back from a socially engaged life is an apparently intolerable idea. The objections move in two directions, scientific and political. Scientifically, it is denied that any strong evidence can be found, in our society or others, to provide support for the supposed universality of disengagement. The aged adjust to their new circumstances by the development of worklike roles which provide different forms of social engagement, not their relinquishment. Some critics of the theory have held that aging has no universal meaning, but that the different self-conceptions of the old will be a function of their social context; and in any event, that the internal meaning of aging for the elderly may be different from that assumed from the outside.

Far more important than the scientific criticisms, which turned up sometimes ambiguous results, were the political and ideological objections.[8] The real trouble with a theory of that kind, its critics held, was the support it lent to the worst kind of ageist stereotyping. It imposed upon the old an image of diminishment and self-denying retreat, and it provided society with an allegedly scientific theory that would allow it to sweetly but still firmly belittle and dismiss the elderly. Disengagement theory was, in short, a view of the elderly utterly incompatible with the then-emerging new agenda of advocacy for the aged. That agenda was to project the process of aging as utterly diverse and individual, the aged as varied (like any other age group), and old age as a time of renewed vigor, growth, self-discovery, and contributions to the community; a time of vigorous engagement, not disengagement.

Just where does that counterattack on disengagement and the modernization which stands behind it leave those ancient, and barely repressed, questions which have ever been part of aging? What does my bodily decline mean, and why must I endure it? Why must my oldest and dearest friends die—"These days I spend most of my time," one man said, "at funerals"—and why, along with them, must I die? If under the new modernized order we are not supposed to disengage to give some concerted time to thinking about such troubling questions, just when and how are we supposed to think about them? In a golf cart between the greens if we are healthy and affluent? Or while sitting uncomfortably and idly on the front steps in the slums if we are poor and arthritic? Or during the ample time for dark thoughts afforded the aged spouse of an aged Alzheimer's victim, who might wonder just what kind of a universe it is that brings some of us so low before blowing us away altogether?

However flawed its empirical basis, disengagement theory tried to make sense of the way the elderly confront limits. That they do not necessarily do so in terms of the kind of disengagement envisioned in the original theory should not distract attention from the importance that dealing with limits can and should play in old age. At the heart of the modernizing project is an attempt to deny limits, to act as if old age could do without them, or could proceed by pretending they do not exist. The value of a sense of limits, however, is not only its realism but also that by providing a boundary, it forces a facing up to the course of a life and to the fact that it exists within a finite length of time. That may be, and usually is, a harsh discipline, but it is a necessary starting point for self-knowledge and for the location of the self within a community that not only coexists with oneself but also is located in the stream of history, among those who went before and those who will come after. A clear-sighted awareness of limits makes possible that kind of understanding. If the recognition of limits is necessary to understand the course and trajectory of one's life, it has some other rewards as well. Ronald Blythe, writing of the later years of D. H. Lawrence, notes that while in most respects he was burned out, he knew how to work within limits: ". . . he enjoyed making something from the ashes, and in this he shared one of the subtle pleasures of the very old, which is the utilization of one's frailty and slightness, the knowing how short a distance one can go—and then going it. The knowing that one need not do more because it is impossible to do more. Ever again."9

The modernization project does not care to deal with the deeply disturbing questions of decline and death.10 They are heavy, unpleasant, not readily compatible with the new, exciting, upbeat kind of aging being sought. But the questions are as real and pressing now as ever, and there ought to be some socially affirmed way of pulling back and regrouping ourselves as individuals to confront our finitude, our bodily dissolution, and our eventual death. While disengagement is probably not the right term or theory, there is good reason to take some degree of withdrawal from the affairs of the world as good, a way of recognizing the ultimate falsity of seeing old age merely as a continuation of earlier stages of life and of relegating the deeply disturbing questions it must bring to the closet of our night selves. Death is a reality, and it deserves time for preparation, not merely for the filing of a "living will." Bodily decline is a reality, and this must be managed and accepted. And despite all the brave words, social disengagement is, save for the extraordinarily lucky few, an eventual reality as well. What Elizabeth Markson has called our "socially obligatory" roles must and will decline and disappear with old age.11 The old can remain economically and socially productive. There the modernizers are perfectly correct. They cannot, however, remain socially *indispensable* in the way that children and younger adults are for a society. It will not escape the eye of the young or old that the young can do, and need to do, most of that which the old once did. Life goes on when the old die, and the world continues to run.

What might be the ingredients of an image of old age that manages, looking in one direction, to incorporate some of the sensible new possibilities for the aging; and, looking in another, to retain from the past of many cultures the valuable idea that old age should be a time for reflective acceptance of decline and preparation for death, for wise but not supine withdrawal? Two preliminary steps seem necessary: that we collectively work toward the creation of (if we cannot rediscover) a social purpose for the aged, and that there be a refurbishing of the ancient idea of life stages. The intent of creating social purpose would be to provide a nourishing setting for the last stage of life; and there exists a need to make something of that last stage in order to give credibility to the social purpose. Yet these preliminary steps are, though necessary, not sufficient conditions for a full-fledged possibility of meaning and significance. They must have a plausible content if they are to carry weight. I will turn first to the preliminary tasks.

| Social Purpose and the Life Cycle

THE ELDERLY WERE OFTEN granted a high status in earlier, more traditional societies because of the belief that age carried with it not only wisdom, but a privileged ability to interpret the moral traditions of a society. For a society like ours which in its secular and public guise professes to have no generally binding moral traditions, this presents an obvious problem. The aged will not have a common moral tradition of which they are a part to pass on to the young, only particular sectarian values and traditions, perhaps useful within tight-knit families but not within society as a whole.[12] This conclusion is even more distressing than it might initially seem. If the aged cannot be a critical link in passing on public tradition—part of which is to serve as the living memory of earlier embodiments and exemplars of some central values and perspectives—then they are left with scarcely any *societal* purpose at all as aged people (however pleasant they may find their lives).

They will not necessarily be ignored. They will be welcomed by business as consumers; by their children as a source of funds, family anecdotes, and occasional baby-sitting; by politicians as active, motivated voters; and by nonprofit agencies as a source of volunteer help to replace the onetime housewives now out in the marketplace. In none of these roles is it their age *as such* that is prized, much less their link to still-viable traditions and older perspectives. It is the accidental features of their age that are attractive: their free time, their disposable income (at least in the case of many), and their eagerness to find something to do with themselves in the absence of obligatory roles. Take away those aspects of the aged population and little of substance is left.

Why should the old not wonder just what their value is in that situation? Why should there be any surprise that efforts to stress their real and potential "contributions" to society often fail to reassure? If those contributions have little if anything to do with what the aged know and can do because they are old and have lived a long life, then they have little to do with what is a central part of being old. That a kind of "busy hands are happy hands" philosophy for the old, in the absence of a core valuation of the old for their own sake, can work as a solution to the profound mysteries of aging and death is at best naive, at worst mischievous.[13] Those features are prized in which they resemble younger age groups, not those which make them *old* people.

This was not always the case. People, in what the historian Thomas Cole has called the late Calvinist tradition of the end of the eighteenth through the early part of the nineteenth century in America, saw old age as the completion of a pilgrimage, a time requiring gravity, vigilance, patience, and resignation, in every way a preparation for death, but also a time of service—by virtue of that very preparation—to family and community. They had a way of integrating their lives into larger belief systems, blending a view of self, community, and the sacred into a unified whole.[14] By the 1850s, a new and by now more familiar ideal began to appear. Where an earlier generation of ministers had urged a wariness about the possibility of a long life, Victorian ministers urged just the opposite: an avoidance of thoughts about death and preparation for a long old age. Health, activity, and usefulness were to be cultivated to the very end. Age was to be mastered rather than accepted, eliminated if possible rather than explored. The increasing dominance of a scientific outlook accelerated a rejection of decline and decay, especially those fundamental forms represented by aging and death.

There quickly followed an emphasis on the virtues of youth rather than age, the new rather than the old, self-reliance and autonomy rather than community. The seeds of the later ageism of the twentieth century were being sown. But while repudiating ageism, we have not rejected those values which stimulated it in the first place. The power of ageism will remain all the more insidious because of the open conspiracy to present old age as a time of continuing zest and discovery. As Thomas Cole concludes, "If old age in America had only suffered the usual misfortune of being identified with an old order, the impact might have been short-lived. But old age not only symbolized the eighteenth-century world of patriarchy and hierarchical authority, it also represented a new embarrassment to the new morality of self-control. The primary virtues of civilized morality [the successor to "late Calvinism"]—independence, health, success—required constant control over one's body and physical energies. The decaying body in old age, a constant reminder of the limits of physical self-control, came to signify dependence, disease, failure, and sin. . . . Old age, too, succumbed to the vacuum of meaning surrounding the end of life. . . . Older people today are encouraged to strive for the physical health and self-control previously attributed to the young and middle-aged. Underneath this vision of ceaseless activity, spurred by the illusory promise of scientifically abolishing biological aging, lies a profound failure of meaning."[15]

Of course, it might be responded that however attractive those earlier days of patriarchy or "late Calvinism" may have been, we no longer live in those times, and they cannot be recovered—even if we cared to pay the price of life in that kind of world, which by no means everyone would. Life in our times, the retort would continue, requires that we learn to live without "meaning," at least the kind of meaning that is grounded in some common social and cosmic order. That we cannot have. Even if painful and lacking in consolation, it might be said, its absence is the price of our freedom, the necessary condition of our pluralism, and a spur to finding within the private self and not within the community a center of psychological gravity and meaning.

That response is inadequate. The fact that we cannot return to an earlier time does not imply the need to repudiate altogether the ideal which undergirded it: that old age has to find an integral place in the lives of those who would and did become old, and that an old age lacking in meaning is not, save for the rarest person, a humanly tolerable condition. Yet even if there is some agreement that the search for a common meaning would be valuable, it requires the complementary help of a reinvigorated theory of the life cycle. One of the most frequently cited, but least analyzed, passages in the literature on aging and the life cycle is from the writings of Erik Erikson: "As we come to the last state [old age], we become aware of the fact that our civilization really does not harbor a concept of the whole of life. . . . Any span of the cycle lived without vigorous meaning, at the beginning, in the middle, or at the end, endangers the sense of life and the meaning of death in all those whose life stages are intertwined."[16]

A slightly more accurate interpretation might be that our civilization has repudiated the concept of the whole of life. This represents a tantalizing but finally nostalgic and dangerous position, one that is a direct rebuke to the modernization project. A concept of a whole life requires a number of conditions we seem reluctant to agree to: (1) that life has relatively fixed stages—a notion rejected on the ground that we are free to make of our different stages of chronological age whatever we want; biology presents no unalterable philosophical and moral constraints or any clear pointers; (2) that death may present an "absolute limit" to life—an idea repudiated because of the ability of medicine to constantly push back the boundary line between life and death; life is an open-ended possibility, not a closed circle; (3) that old age is of necessity marked by decline and thus requires a unique set of meanings to take account of that fact—a viewpoint that must be rejected as part of the political struggle against ageism, which would make of the old a deviant, marginal, and burdensome group; and (4) that "our civilization" would be better off if it shared some common view of "the whole of life"—rejected as a politically hazardous notion, more congenial to authoritarian and collectivist cultures than to those marked by moral and religious pluralism and individualism.

A similar fate has overcome some of Erikson's important insights into old age as the final stage of life. By his emphasis on integrity (by which he means coherence and wholeness) as the most desirable trait of old age, he implicitly highlights the finality of that stage, the need to bring life to a close in a thoughtful fashion. Yet integrity, he realizes, is still too general a concept, and requires a more specific focus in the aged, that of "wisdom," by which he means an "informed and detached concern with life itself in the face of death itself."[17] Erikson is well aware that old age in our day is different, marked by much longer lives for more people. Still, he asks "should historical changes dissuade us from what we have once perceived old age to be, in our own lifetime and according to the distilled knowledge that has survived in folk wit as well as in folk wisdom?"[18] His answer is no, although he agrees that some adjustments will be needed. Instead ". . . a historical change like the lengthening of the average life span calls for viable reritualizations, which must provide a meaningful interplay between beginning and end as well as some finite sense of summary and, possibly, a more active anticipation of dying. For all this, *wisdom* will still be a valid word—and so, we think, will *despair*."[19]

| The Construction of Meaning

OUT OF WHAT CLOTH can the old cut integrity, wisdom, and meaning? Erikson hints at an answer by affirming that old age ought not to represent a repudiation of the earlier adult stage of generativity, encompassing as it did procreativity, productivity, and creativity.[20] It must now take a different, more capacious, form—what he calls a "*grand*-generative function."[21] Erikson provides few details about what that might consist of other than to say, all too vaguely, that it will require a kind of "vital involvement."[22] The problem is that in the face of modernization, the involvement must be much different from and richer than the kind of vigorous and vital carrying-on, more-of-the-same, open-ended, meaning-evasive philosophy which is by now its standard version. As a general specification, it must fully acknowledge the vitality built on better health and more years that are now part of ordinary old age and open to still more modification in the future. It must no less acknowledge that life is still finite and time-limited, bounded as ever by death and usually still preceded by a decline of many vital capacities. It is still a stage of life shot through with loss and desperately requiring that sense be made of it, that its mysteries and terrors be confronted.

Various sources of meaning and significance are available for the aged, each still possible and each still needed. Time will provide me with a metaphor as I try to suggest what they might be. The elderly are in the best position to keep alive the *past*, to integrate the history of which they are a living link with that present which they share with younger generations. This could be as valuable in our society as it was in preliterate societies. The integration of what was and what is, and how they cohere with each other, is something that only the elderly can provide within the confines of family and local community life. Only they are in a position to have experienced some patterns and cycles; the young tend to think they saw the dawn of history. The various movements to encourage the elderly to recapture their own pasts, and to make them available to the young, is a healthy recognition of the value of that role. It is both their unique privilege and their unique obligation.

The aged are exceedingly well placed to appreciate what it means to live in the *present*. Their future is foreshortened, and unlike the young, they are not as a rule preparing themselves to be something other than they already are. What they have today is all they have. Even if there is a tomorrow, and a day after that, it will pass all too quickly. Making the most of today is an art which a person of any age can cultivate, and an old person is compelled to cultivate. That much old age is now accompanied by some degree of chronic illness makes the task both more necessary and more complicated: the mind must be distracted, the limitations framed and domesticated, and the present—in whatever form it presents itself—enjoyed or at least made the most of.[23]

The aged bear a particular obligation to the *future*, and it is that aspect I most want to dwell on here. Not only is it the most neglected perspective on the elderly, but it is the most pertinent as we try to understand the problem of their health care. The young—children and young adults—most justly and appropriately spend their time preparing for future roles and developing a self pertinent to them. The mature adult has the responsibility to procreate and rear the next generation and to manage the present society. What can the elderly most appropriately do? It should be the special role of the elderly to be the moral conservators of that which has been and the most active proponents of that which will be after they are no longer here. Their indispensable role as conservators is what generates what I believe ought to be the *primary* aspiration of the old, which is to serve the young and the future. Just as they were once the heirs of a society built by others, who passed on to them what they needed to know to keep it going, so are they likewise obliged to do the same for those who will follow them.

Only the old—who alone have seen in their long lives first a future on the horizon and then its actual arrival—can know what it means to go from past through present to future. That is valuable and unique knowledge. If the young are to flourish, then the old should step aside in an active way, working until the very end to do what they can to leave behind them a world hopeful for the young and worthy of bequest. The acceptance of their aging and death will be the principal stimulus to doing this. It is this seemingly paradoxical combination of withdrawal to prepare for death and an active, helpful leave-taking oriented toward the young which provides the possibility for meaning and significance in a contemporary context. Meaning is provided because there is a purpose in that kind of aging, combining an identity for the self with the serving of a critical function in the lives of others—that of linking the past, present, and future—something which, even if they are unaware of it, they cannot do without. Significance is provided because society, in recognizing and encouraging the aged in their duties toward the young, gives them a clear and important role, one that both is necessary for the common good and that *only* they can play.

| Aspirations to Serve the Young

Is IT EVEN NECESSARY to stress service to the young as an aspiration of the old? Is it not true that even now, the elderly are a prime resource, through the family, to the young? That is perfectly true and should not be forgotten. The elderly already provide everything from child care (some 17 percent of the care of children of working mothers is provided by grandparents), to living space, to supplementary and emergency income, to advice for younger family members.[24] In fragmented families they are often the only source of unity and stability. The family remains the most important mechanism for income redistribution, and there is evidence to suggest that within the family, the elderly may give more assistance than they receive.[25] The importance of the elderly in the lives of families is, then, as vital as it is undeniable. Family life would be immeasurably poorer without their contributions.

Yet it would be a serious mistake to think that, as important as they are, service and sacrifice within the context of the family can suffice to provide either full meaning or significance for the aged. Meaning is enhanced by a sense of obligation to other age groups and a linkage to other generations. The elderly, if they want to find a larger meaning, need to serve the young in the larger, public society as well.[26] Not all will be able physically to do this, but many will. A contribution in the private sphere of the family is not tantamount to service to the public welfare, even if the latter requires such service for its own flourishing. The money that family members may give each other is not the same as the payment of taxes or voluntary activities to help other people's children; each serves important, but different, ends. (A similar point should be made about younger people. They need to develop, early in life, their own feelings of obligation to those still younger—not only their siblings, but others as well.)

There is another important distinction to be made. Many services and benefits provided within families by the old are not of a kind that only an older person could provide; again, it is usually a case of the older person's having available time or disposable income, something that others could in principle provide. In saying this, I do not mean to minimize or belittle that kind of assistance. It counts for much and bespeaks a considerable reservoir of affection and devotion between young and old within families. It does not, however, wholly meet the criteria I believe central—the discovery of a place for the old in their own minds and in that of society which they, and only they, can take precisely because they are aged. The provision of advice and counsel to younger friends and family members comes closest to what I have in mind; that is where the age and experience do count. There is, then, a painful irony here. If we had a better system of social services—income maintenance, home care for chronically ill or injured children and young adults, child-care facilities—then there would be much less need for the many things that older family members now of necessity do for younger ones. Their role would diminish and might be adequately performed by others. In that respect, some of the present roles of the elderly within families are valuable but not irreplaceable. The elderly need a more solid footing in the life of the community than that.

What is it that *only* the old can provide the young, that which is irreplaceable in their contribution? *Only* the aged can provide a perspective the young need if they are properly to envision their own lives: that of the cycle of the generations and its import for the living of a life. The young may be indifferent to that perspective; the elderly may have to struggle to make it known. What the old know, though too poignantly at times perhaps, is that the generations come and go and that time unceasingly marches on, and on, and on, all too soon passing us all by. For the very young, the sole world they know or can well imagine is the present world in which they exist. Time for them usually moves too slowly, withholding the freedoms and self-realizations they long for. The past is little more than an illusion, something to be found in history books, not in their memories. In one sense, time will cure their problem; it will march on for them also. In another sense, they need the old to give them a perspective they desperately, if unknowingly, require while still young, that of the need to visualize their life as a whole, to see where they are going, to be helped to know where they ought to be going, to be given a prod toward asking early on what they would like, when the end has come, to have made of themselves and to be remembered for.

As Alasdair MacIntyre has written of the moral life: ". . . both childhood and old age have [mistakenly] been wrenched from the rest of human life and made over into distinct realms. . . . it is the distinctiveness of each and not the unity of the life of the individual . . . of which we are taught to think and to feel. . . . The unity of a human life [should instead be] the unity of a narrative quest."[27] The notion of a "narrative quest," MacIntyre reminds us, requires that we have some conception of a goal, a *telos,* toward which the quest works; it requires both self-knowledge and a sense of the nature of the good that is sought. The good in this case, I propose, is that of providing the young with an image of the pursuit of a life of meaning.

Both the old and the young turn out to need the same thing: a way of imaginatively and reflectively integrating their individual life stages into the larger cycle of the generations. The young are not in a position to do this well for themselves. They ordinarily have neither the experience nor the seasoned sensibilities necessary to do so. Only the old can bring them to it. The young, in that respect, need the old to help them discover their own sense of meaning (just as the young, for their part, need to do it for those still younger than they). At the same time, it is the provision of that kind of meaning to the young which ought to be the greatest source of meaning for the old themselves. None but they in a society can do that. There is no substitute for age in that kind of quest, as there can be if only money is needed, or help with child care. By this kind of service to the young, by this construction of a world of meaning, the old turn out to be benefiting not only the present welfare of the young, but also, and simultaneously, their future welfare—and, even more, the welfare of still another generation after that, for they are tacitly instructing the young and middle-aged in what they should begin doing with the generation that is to succeed them.

What I am saying requires two assumptions. The young must be prepared to look among the old for models, and the old should be willing to see themselves in the service of future generations in general, not only the welfare of their own children and grandchildren in particular. There is no way to ensure that the young will look to the old; but there are some grounds for thinking that the chances are greater now than in the past: the increasing proportion of the aged, making them more visible and more present as a daily reality and as people the young will personally know; the better health of the aged, enhancing the likelihood they will be more active in the community; and the possibility that, as the aged increasingly contemplate their own role, they will see the value of working toward the future of the young and of providing a model for them as an attractive one. As for the possibility that the old will come to that last perception, I can only try to sketch here some reasons why they should, hoping that their own need to find meaning for themselves, and the need of society to reconstitute and find significance for their social status, will provide a helpful prod.

The unique capacity of the elderly to see the way past, present, and future interact provides the foundation for the contribution they can make to the young and to future generations. "Society," Edmund Burke wrote in *Reflections on the Revolution in France,* is a "partnership not only between those who are living, but between those who are living, those who are dead and those who are to be born."[28] That may be perfectly true; but why should the old, who will be passing from the scene, have any motivation to continue that partnership or feel they have any special contribution to make to it? They should know that they have their own debt to the past and that from that debt springs their own obligation to the future. The best retort to the old and cynical query "What has posterity ever done for me?" is that it can and will judge us for what we left it. If we value our own life at all, then we should value and feel some obligation toward those who made that life possible, our own families and the past societies which supported them. We owe to those coming after us at least what we were given by those who came before us, the possibility of life and survival. We also owe to the future an amelioration of those conditions which, in our own life, lessened our possibilities of living a decent life and which, if they persist, will do the same for coming generations. If the aged, moreoever, want to find meaning in their lives, and a significant place in society, then this is their most promising direction, drawing on that which only they can give.

There is a necessary biological and social link between the generations; later generations exist because of burdens assumed by earlier generations. This is most evident in the case of close successor generations. The later requires the earlier. It is no less present even when the generations are separated over time. To live at all is to be linked in an inextricable way to the past, and to be no less a powerful determinant of the fate of future generations. That is what the aged can see, and that is what they can pass on to the young.

Even more can be said, a still more powerful motivation invoked. It may be only through passing life and culture along to the next generation—in an active and responsible and yet gradually self-emptying way—that any kind of transcendence can be found. Leon Kass has written suggestively that ". . . biology has its own view of our nature and its inclinations. Biology also teaches about transcendence, though it eschews talk about the soul. For self-preservation is one thing, reproduction quite another; in bearing and caring for their young, many animals risk and even sacrifice their own lives. Indeed, in all higher animals, to reproduce *as such* implies both acceptance of the death of self and participation in its transcendence. . . . human biology, too, teaches us how our life points beyond itself—to our offspring, to our community, to our species. Man, like the other animals, is built for reproduction. Man, more than the other animals, is also built for sociality. And man, alone among the animals, is built for culture—not only through capacities to transmit and receive skills and techniques, but also through capacities for shared beliefs, opinions, rituals, traditions."[29]

| Obligations and Virtues

THE MODERNIZERS OF AGING, I suppose, might have a retort to my particular projection of a role for the elderly. They might say that, to the extent the old (say, the "young-old") are still in good health and vigorous in their outlook, they should be allowed to relinquish the burdens of responsibility to the young; they do not need "transcendence" so much as an opportunity to cultivate their own fulfillment during their last years. Have they not done enough already? Can they not be allowed at last to live for themselves? If they are in addition already ill or disabled is it not naive to expect of them much more than survival? How can they be expected to serve younger generations, and why should that weight be added to the weights imposed by their years?

That viewpoint deserves some sympathy, but it also presents a dilemma. If the old are to have meaning in their own lives and significance in the larger social world, they cannot claim a right to self-absorption or an exemption from civic duties. Those same forces of modernization which would have them pretend that aging does not occur, or can with sufficient energy be brought to heel, work against giving the aged their own unique and valued role. This can be achieved only through recognition that old age is the last phase of life, that it cannot go on for long, and that death is on its way. But aging as a stage of life can be given a meaning equal in value to earlier stages only if it is understood as requiring every bit as much vigor, dedication, and imagination as those earlier stages. Gruman has argued that only *more* modernization will suffice to bring to completion the modernization project now under way; we cannot, in his view, stop now without risking the loss of what we already have. I want to argue, by way of repudiating this project, that it is only through toughly and energetically embracing old age as a time of both service to the future and decline and withdrawal that its value as a stage in life can ultimately be redeemed.

It is grace under adversity that can impress the young, not the ability of the old to pretend they are still young. It will be the political skills and voting-participation rates turned to the service of the young that will commend the old to the young and to future generations, not the search for their own security. It will be the wisdom of the old—that old-fashioned, supposedly anachronistic virtue—which will, if the old work to cultivate their perceptions, catch the ear of the young—not the street smarts of the old in knowing how to survive in a world of young people. The dilemma of the old, in sum, cannot be resolved except by their taking the harder, more demanding role, one that will not allow them to let up, or be excused, because of their age; or allow them, through the modernizing impulse, to reject aging altogether.

How are we to strike the right balance here? To age with grace is to accept decline and loss, to accept the reality that one's life is coming to an end, to understand that a final attempt must be made to make sense of oneself and one's place in relation to those who went before and those who will come after. This need not be a wholly passive self-examination, or preclude an active engagement in the life around one; "disengagement" can be understood in an active sense. The great danger is self-absorption, the embracing of service to self or the "rewarding" of oneself as a way of warding off, or attempting to compensate for, the death that is to come. The common phrase that "it is my turn" manifests this tendency. Two writers, at a great historical remove from each other, have addressed that danger, but in different ways.

Simone de Beauvoir wrote in *The Coming of Age*: "The greatest good fortune, even greater than health, for the old person is to have his world inhabited by projects; then, busy and useful, he escapes both from boredom and from decay. . . . There is only one solution if old age is not to be an absurd parody of our former life, and that is to go on pursuing ends that give our existence a meaning—devotion to individuals, to groups or to causes, social, political, intellectual or creative work. In spite of the moralists' opinion to the contrary, in old age we should still wish to have passions strong enough to prevent us turning in upon ourselves."[30] Harry R. Moody has characterized this passage as one displaying "an activist style of growing old. . . . Old age, in this view, is not a time for wisdom or summing up. It is a time for continual engagement."[31] I am less certain about how this passage should be understood. Nothing that Mme. de Beauvoir says need be rejected by one who believes that the most important aspect of growing old should be a focus on larger questions of meaning; this does not preclude an active concern about the world one is soon to leave. But if the "turning in" that de Beauvoir would have us avoid is meant to evade these questions, then it will be a mistake.

Cicero, writing in 44 B.C., strikes a different note. While the old should see their physical labors reduced, their mental and social activities should actually increase. "Old men . . . as they become less capable of physical exertion, should redouble their intellectual activity, and their principal occupation should be to assist the young, their friends, and above all their country with their wisdom and sagacity. There is nothing they should guard against so much as languor and sloth. Luxury, which is shameful at every period of life, makes old age hideous. If it is united with sensuality, the evil is two-fold. Age thus brings disgrace on itself and aggravates the shameless license of the young."[32] The combination of a rejection of old age as a time for self-indulgence, the astute observation that the old can provide poor models of morality for the young if they are not careful, and the idea of service to the larger community suggests dimensions in the understanding of old age of a kind wider than those of de Beauvoir.

For our own time, we need just those virtues which Cicero stressed. To complement an ethos that for well over two decades now has stressed the rights and entitlements of the elderly, there would be one which held them up to high standards of service and stewardship, and did so because of their important and indispensable contributions which could not otherwise be realized.[33] William F. May has written that "Any serious reflection on the moral status of the aged requires reflection on the specific virtues that age calls for." "Such discussion," he cautions, "will deteriorate into the sentimental if we do not remind ourselves that virtues hardly come automatically with age; rather, they are structures of character that come with resolution, prayer, suffering, and persevering."[34] Among the virtues he lists are *courage* in the face of certain decline and death; *humility* in response to progressive loss and the humiliation of body and dignity that it can bring; *patience* out of a need to take control of oneself when the loss of control begins to gain sway; *simplicity* as a way of traveling light; *benignity* (a kind of "purified benevolence") to offset tendencies to avarice, possessiveness, and manipulation; and (most surprisingly) *hilarity* ". . . a celestial gaiety in those who have seen a lot, done a lot, grieved a lot, but now acquire that detachment of the fly on the ceiling looking down on the human scene."[35] To this list I would add *vigor of spirit*, by which I mean the drive to keep going to carry out one's hope to serve the young, an impulse of dogged determination to work to the very end for a future one will not see. None of this is to deny that the elderly can become tired, can feel a strong need to pull away from the fray of life. That should be their right if they can bear no more. Yet one may be allowed to hope that however diminished the body, the mind and spirit will struggle on.

3 | Medicine and the Conquest of Aging

As a human enterprise, medicine appears to be one of the most organized and purposive. It is a bustling, ambitious, exciting, and frequently noble drama. The conquest of illness and disease, the relief of pain, and the forestalling of death are its generally recognized goals. Yet that view conveys a unity of effort that is, in reality, something more coherent than the truth of the matter. Little thought is given in medicine to its ultimate ends. It is more like an ensemble of piecework than the creation of an integrated tapestry. Here there are researchers working on cancer, there on arthritis, and over there on Alzheimer's disease. Others pursue molecular genetics, and still others the dynamic of the central nervous system. Researchers go where their interests carry them, or where the money for research can be found, or where the clamor for results is most powerful. Just what this is meant to come to in the long run is not clear, nor is that of great interest in its day-to-day work. Sufficient unto the day, it seems to say, are the present evils of illness and disease.

This kind of medical pluralism surely promotes vigor and diversity of effort. But the time has come in the case of medicine and the care of the aging to develop a more purposive agenda, one that asks just what it is we are after. The short-term successes of medicine continue to divert attention from the now-recognized cumulative social burdens of an aging society they are creating, and no less from the change in meaning and expectation that has been elicited about getting old. We can no longer afford to avert our eyes from what that signifies. Two basic questions need now to be posed. How should we specify and pursue the appropriate goals of medicine in light of the new possibilities of aging as a stage of life? The second question is the converse of the first: how should we specify the meaning and role of aging in light of the new possibilities of medicine?

I want to argue that medicine should be used not for the further extension of the life of the aged, but only for the full achievement of a natural and fitting life span and thereafter for the relief of suffering. At the same time, we need to clarify the goals of aging. The primary aspirations of the old should include, among their own reasonable needs, the needs of their fellow elderly and of their families, as well as the welfare of the young in general and of the coming generations. The complementary goal of medicine should be to help the aged maintain a physical and psychological life sufficient to enhance the realization of those aspirations; that is, not more life as such, but a life free of whatever pain and suffering might impede these ends. While the question of resource allocation provides an occasion to inquire into the relationship between the goals of medicine and the future of aging (see Chapter 5), I do not intend to rest my case on that basis, even though it provides some collateral support. I want to lay the foundation for a more austere thesis: that even with relatively ample resources, there will be better ways in the future to spend our money than on indefinitely extending the life of the elderly. That is neither a wise social goal nor one that the aged themselves should want, however compellingly it will attract them.

Medicine in its daily practice has historically paid little attention to the process of aging and its inevitable outcome, death. There has, to be sure, been a long-standing theoretical interest in the biological causes of aging and death and in the relationship of disease to those causes. There has been no less an interest, particularly of late, in how the medical needs of the elderly might best be met. What I mean is that clinical medicine has not tried specifically to define its purpose in relation to the process of aging as the final stage of the life process. It has instead directed its attention to resisting death and to the treatment of diseases regardless of the age of those who contract them. It has thus been notably age-egalitarian, and it is still common for most physicians to resist the idea that the age of a patient might count against giving that patient beneficial care. Behind that attitude is the ancient moral principle that the ill should be treated, whatever their own circumstances or the nature of their illness. That "beneficial" care will be understood differently perhaps, dependent upon age and other patient conditions and characteristics, need not tell against the widespread acceptance of that general principle. There is an important difference between taking age into account in order to provide the most appropriate treatment and the use of age as a standard for the discriminatory denial or modification of treatment.

The historical context of the development of the principle of an age-blind standard of treatment was that of the long period of medical and human history which saw death as a common occurrence at all stages of life, and the attainment of old age the good fortune of a small percentage only. As Ronald Blythe has nicely put it, ". . . we place dying in what we take to be its logical position, which is at the close of a long life, whereas our ancestors accepted the futility of placing it in any position at all. In the midst of life we are in death, they said, and they meant it. To them it was a fact; to us it is a metaphor."[1] In early New England during the seventeenth century, for instance, only some 4 to 7 percent of the population was over the age of 60, with between 10 and 14 percent of the adult population over that age.[2] With the high infant-mortality rate of pre-industrial societies, the large number of women who died in childbirth, and the great prevalence of deadly infectious diseases which struck down those of all ages, there was little reason to single out for attention the special causes of illness and death of the elderly. Not many people got that far. While the notion of a "premature death" as a target of medical energy has a modern ring to it, the idea has long been present in medicine. It was generally construed to mean death prior to old age, and "old age" was earlier understood in Anglo-American society to begin by the late 50s or early 60s. Any extended life after that time was simply good fortune. Death beyond that point was not a premature end to be fought with any urgency by medicine.

Two features of contemporary medicine have changed that situation. The first is the conquest of most infectious diseases and the second, the great reduction in infant mortality. Together, they all but ensure that most people will live past the age of 65; 85 percent of women already do survive that long.[3] While that hardly means medicine has lost or will lose interest in the pathologies affecting younger generations (as the advent of neonatal medicine and organ transplantation amply demonstrates), it does mean that the major new frontiers of medicine are now those conditions which predominantly kill or cripple older people, and as time goes on, older and older people. Young people die of cancer (it is the second leading cause of death among children), but as the correlation of its incidence with the extension of the average life span suggests, it is now more characteristically a disease of the old, as are heart diseases and stroke. The ongoing "war" against those diseases will affect the future health and longevity of the elderly much more decisively than any other group. The recently intensified efforts to find genetic markers capable of predicting the likelihood of late-onset disease, such as predisposition to heart disease, generate excitement because of their implications for older rather than younger people. More or less inadvertently—but nonetheless inevitably—the future of biomedical research is going to be a future heavily directed toward the welfare of the elderly; that is, it will be so directed to the extent that forestalling death or ameliorating the symptoms and effects of chronic disease remains its primary goals.

The second feature of contemporary medicine is a consequence of the first: the subtle but inexorable shift in notions and concepts of health, illness, and "premature" death as they apply to the elderly. Part of the shift is attributable to greater scientific knowledge, particularly now that many conditions once thought inherent in old age, such as hearing loss and skeletal fragility, are in fact relatively curable or controllable. Discoveries of that kind have encouraged a more aggressive research agenda for diseases affecting the elderly. That certain conditions are more common or predominant among the old does not prove, many researchers in effect argue, that they need be accepted as inherent in the aging process or as the inevitable fate of all, or even most, of the elderly. They can be pursued simply as remediable conditions, much as one would pursue harmful maladies that afflict younger age groups.

It is but a small step from that mode of thinking, marked by inveterate optimism and a faith in aggressive scientific research, to a shift in the criteria for "premature" death (or, for that matter, premature debilities more generally). At present, for example, the Centers for Disease Control classifies "premature mortality" in terms of "years of potential life lost"; that is, as "a measure of premature mortality over the arbitrary span from the first birthday until completion of the 64th year of life."[4] But note that the obviously conventional time scope of that definition is called "arbitrary," and there is no doubt that many would agree with the use of that phrase. The use of age 65 as the dividing line for Social Security as well as for many other standard indications of the advent of old age is, after all, a legacy of the nineteenth century, where it was first used in the German social security system established by Bismarck. From that perspective, the choice of age 65 as the criterion of "premature" death is obviously historically conditioned; and as medical history moves on, any age might be seen as arbitrary. In 1900, people lived an average of twelve years beyond 65; now they live some seventeen years. In a decade, they may live still another few years longer.

This otherwise encouraging trend is deeply troubling from another perspective. It provides a decent basis neither for specifying the goals of medicine in the care of the elderly nor for developing a public policy that can allocate fairly between the generations. If concepts such as "old," "aging," and "premature death" are a function of the state-of-the-art of medicine at any given moment, then it is hard to imagine a solid basis for determining what health demands, expectations, or desires on the part of the elderly are reasonable or unreasonable (or what count as fair expectations of the young about their health as they age).

But even if we cannot achieve great precision, some lines must be drawn, some way found of making some meaningful distinctions. Contemporary medical theory and practice offer little help in this respect. The indifference of medicine to distinguishing sharply between medical needs and desires, and no less its working relativism about what goods might properly be hoped for in the name of health, become manifest when questions about the ends of medicine and aging are raised. That trait is, however, perfectly compatible with the focus on individual well-being that has provided an undeniable impetus to medical research. There is, I think, a tacit moral premise that sustains the support and celebrity of contemporary medicine: unless there is some immediately visible harm that can be proved, then we are all free under the expansive aegis of medical progress to pursue any personal vision at all of good health and life purposes. The shortcomings of that underlying ideology, otherwise so attractively permissive and expansive of choice, become nowhere more evident than in trying to decide what we should, as a society, seek for the elderly and, when we ourselves become elderly, what we should wisely seek for ourselves. Of course we want our old people to lead lives of dignity, and part of that dignity lies in the well-founded hope that one's old age will be respected.

But just what should the old, and those of us who will become old, hope for from medicine? If life is so good, should we expect medicine always to resist the aging process and the diseases that finally bring about death? Many would say yes. But perhaps some people will want to give up. Should medicine be no less willing to accommodate itself to their wishes? The common answer to that question is a yes also. Should not we each, that is, be free to do what we want so long as that poses no obvious harm to others? Should we not in the same vein also be free to devise our own meanings for "health" and "disease," simply as a way of recognizing that with medical advances, reality is not fixed but is malleable to our hopes and needs?

A response to those questions requires coming directly to grips with some difficult issues. We need to know whether we should seek some collective agreement on the goals of medicine and the care of the aged, or leave that problem to the uninhibited operation of the individualistic marketplace of money, ideas, and desires. We also need to know whether we can find some meanings of "old age," "health," and "illness" that are not solely artifacts of the passing state of medical research and art but can be grounded in an understanding of the proper ends of medicine. We no less need to know whether we can find some characterization of "premature death" that can be rooted in a solid understanding of human life and whether, in that respect, it makes any sense now to speak of a "natural life span" and a "tolerable death." If we could find plausible solutions to those problems, we would be in a much stronger position to devise suitable long-term goals for medicine in its stance toward the elderly.

| Individualism, Aging, and Health Care

I WANT TO DEAL QUICKLY, and surely inadequately, with the first issue, since the question of individualism is much too large to be explored here. Individualism, and the classical political liberalism of the eighteenth and nineteenth centuries upon which it is based, rests upon the right of individuals to seek that which in their private judgment will bring them happiness. The only limit upon that right is that they may not do harm to others in seeking their personal self-fulfillment. This view has sometimes recently been referred to as a "thin theory" of the human good; that is, it does not rest upon a substantive theory or belief about just what is ultimately good for human beings or ultimately good for society.[5] It has no such underlying theory and remains silent about whether a defensible one is even possible. The search for the good of human life, for its purposes and ends and meaning (if any), is left to the individual. The search for the good is not, and must not become, a collective enterprise to be pursued by the community as a whole, much less by the state.

An equivalent thin theory of aging and health care would say something more or less like the following. Individual people will look upon aging in different ways, express different tolerances for the burdens of old age, seek different goals and lifestyles in old age, and differ about how long they want to live and about the medical conditions under which they are willing to die. It is perfectly fitting in a pluralistic society—one dedicated to individual liberty and opposed to a coerced notion of a good life—that such differences should exist and be allowed to flourish. Medicine should serve that diversity, which does not in any case admit of a single right answer about what people ought to want. Save for evidence that satisfying the desires of some, or many, for a longer and healthy life would do harm to others (surely a difficult fact to establish), medicine should give people what they want. And what do they want? Simply life and good health, themselves perfectly traditional goals even if variously interpreted.

That is a powerful philosophy for the provision of health care, all the more because it makes the values in medicine consistent with the kinds of freedom available in other parts of the society. Yet it also assumes we can afford to leave some basic questions publicly unanswered and unasked. Just what is good for us as we age? What should we hope for? What is the human meaning of old age? The mounting problem of providing health care for the elderly in the setting of an ever-expanding scientific frontier, limited resources, and the inexorable demography of an aging society shows the limitations of a thin theory. Medicine cannot give every person what he or she may desire. Lacking a direction, goals cannot be set. Lacking a deep purpose, coherence cannot be found. Rational priorities can then not be set, or sensible principles of allocation devised. Even within the terms of conventional individualism, there is good reason to believe that satisfying all the desires of the elderly for health care and life extension can do harm to the health needs of other groups and to social needs other than health, such as education, housing, and public transportation. Unlike those of younger age groups, the needs of the elderly for continuing good health are of their very nature open-ended: in old age, the conquest of one disease only guarantees death from some other disease, one which, if conquered, will give way to some further lethal condition. As our present experience demonstrates, the logic of a medical progress set to conquer all disease—in combination with a growing proportion of elderly people—guarantees an ever-rising budget and ever more ways of spending more money. In the absence of unlimited resources, therefore, some degree of harm to other groups must be an inevitable outcome even in the face of efforts to deny the existence of a problem or to imagine a utopian solution.

There is another thin theory which is no less harmful, one that has nothing to do with resources. The price we pay for our individualism in an aging society is that our culture provides neither the elderly nor anyone else with a clear picture of what they should be able to hope for from society in their old age or of the way they might make social sense of their illnesses and eventual death. Given the great importance of meaning for the aged—meaning in their lives and about their place and value in society—there is a harm in the implicit relativism of the diversity itself. There is at present no meaning for the aged unless they can supply it for themselves. Where there should be a public conception of the nature of a good life for the elderly in their weakness and not just in their strength—including the significance of the decline of the body—there is mainly a void. It may be, in fact, that our present, supposedly neutral thin theory actually coerces the elderly by social pressure, particularly in the direction of a forced acceptance of youthful vigor as the ideal of old age.[6] When one sort of aging and death is deemed as good in principle as another, all are increasingly deprived of significance. That some form of rationing of expensive high-technology medicine may be necessary provides still another reason to look for a greater social consensus than a thin theory would countenance. A capricious method of allocation, or one unjustly based on wealth alone, would clearly do harm to many. Even a system that tried to act more fairly (but still had to set some limits) would do harm to the self-worth of the aged unless based on some solidly accepted, dignity-enhancing consensus. Individualism should, in sum, give way to a community-based and affirmed notion of the value of the aged in society and, with that, an acceptance of limits to health care for the aged and medical research of benefit to them. That requires a thick, not a thin, theory of the good.

Medicine is perhaps the last and purest bastion of Enlightenment dreams, tying together reason, science, and the dream of unlimited human possibilities. There is nothing, it is held, that in principle cannot be done and, given suitable caution, little that ought not to be done. Nature, including the body, is seen as infinitely manipulable and plastic to human contrivance. When that conception of medicine is set in the social context of an individualism which is, in principle, opposed to a public consensus about any ultimate human good, it is a potent engine of endless, never-satisfied progress. Yet such a consensus about the human good at least of medicine and aging is exactly what the management of an aging society and of health care for the aged requires. Both the welfare of the elderly for their own sake and the need to allocate resources in some rational and moral way demand that medicine have a clear direction and purpose.

| Aging and the Ends of Medicine

CAN WE, HOWEVER, find within the history and tradition of medicine the resources for a deeper, more rounded, more satisfying account? Leon Kass, in *Toward a More Natural Science,* has provided the most thoughtful and sensitive of recent efforts to grasp and articulate the ends of medicine and the meaning of health, one whose explicit purpose is to set some limits to the enterprise of medicine.

The "end of medicine," Kass argues, is simply that of "health," not the satisfying of wishes, even reasonable ones.[7] Beyond merely capricious wishes, however, happiness and moral virtue—otherwise perfectly valid human goals—are no less outside the legitimate scope of medicine. More surprisingly, he contends that the prolongation of life, or the prevention of death, is also a "false goal" of medicine.[8] Kass is well aware how odd that may sound and explains his point by noting that "*to be alive* and *to be healthy* are not the same," and that "the prolongation of life is ultimately an impossible, or rather an unattainable, goal for medicine. For we are all born with those twin and inescapable 'diseases,' aging and mortality."[9] If physicians can restore a patient's health, it is not medicine but the patient who keeps himself alive; and when health cannot be restored, then death will come. Noting that it is legitimate for medicine to seek to reduce premature deaths (while wryly noting that all deaths seem now to be treated that way), he also contends that, in any case, "medicine's contribution to longer life has nearly reached its natural limit."[10] We should be interested in the "killer" diseases because they are the causes of unhealth rather than because they are killers.[11]

What is "health," such that it, rather than preventing death, should be the goal of medicine? According to Kass, health is bodily wholeness, "or working-well of the work done by the body of a man,"[12] with both subjective and objective manifestations, admitting of degrees (as Aristotle noted) without thereby being indeterminate.[13] "Health" is, therefore, "a natural standard or norm—not a moral norm, not a 'value' as opposed to a 'fact,' . . . the well-working of the organism as a whole."[14] The attractiveness of this approach to health is that not only does it encompass what physicians do in their ordinary clinical work, which is attempt to restore function and thus wholeness to the sick. It also underscores what we note about ourselves when we are ill, that we are not ourselves and that the balances and integrations which mark the ordinary functioning of our body are missing.

For all its attractions, however, the inadequacies of a theory of health limited to wholeness become apparent as soon as we try to apply it to an understanding of medicine's possible role in the face of aging. When, for instance, should a doctor cease trying to restore the wholeness of the body? Or researchers cease trying to cure those diseases which destroy wholeness? There is nothing in Kass's analysis to suggest answers to these questions. Even if one accepts death as an event inherent in biological and human life, it is simply not the case that the prolongation of life is an "impossible" and "unattainable" goal of medicine. Perhaps if "impossible" refers to the possibility of bodily immortality, that may be true. But if a more limited sense is meant, that of a gradual increase in average life expectancy, prolongation has been sought, and with considerable success, throughout the history of medicine, especially during the past century. The motive need not be a desire for bodily immortality, but can simply be part of an incremental quest for a little more life, and then a little more after that, and so on indefinitely. The goal of medicine in practice, whether articulated or not, appears to be to move the wholeness along the continuum of time, not accepting as a given that the wholeness must end in the 60s (as was expected in the eighteenth century), or the 70s (as was expected in the early twentieth century), or the 80s (as we now expect at the end of this century).

Kass is correct in noting that the wholeness of the body is not static when the body is considered in its own right; it is an active process of interaction and integration within. But neither is bodily wholeness a static process over historical time, as medical advances obviously indicate. The body interacts with its environment, one that could be and has been cleansed of lethal bacteria and other pathogens (or protection against them devised) and that is now graced by high-technology medicine. Quite apart from radical high-technology interventions to stave off death, the very type of regimen Kass recommends—one of the promotion of good health habits and personal responsibility for health—has shown itself capable of moving the disintegration of the natural wholeness of the body further along the continuum, that much closer to an average life span of 90 to 100. That outcome could not have been known with any certainty a century ago.

We now increasingly hear also of people living to be 105 or even 110. Why should we not see them, in the name of bodily wholeness, as forerunners of still another leap forward, just as those rare people in their 90s a century ago could have been seen as forerunners of a much larger, and fast-growing group now? If an organ transplant or open-heart surgery is, moreover, an acceptable way to restore wholeness for someone aged 30, why should it be any less acceptable for someone aged 90? Perhaps we cannot, as a society, afford to pay for that kind of life extension, or perhaps we would not be wise to spend our money that way even if we could afford to do so, or perhaps (as Kass also argues) the social disruption of greater life extension cannot socially be borne. But that is a very different way of proceeding than to use the idea of the preservation of health as a way of making the case against unceasing efforts to give the old just a little more life (and then a little more after that, and then still a little more . . .).

I come to this conclusion with considerable regret. It would be salutary to medicine, and to the education of physicians, to be able to find in the idea of health as wholeness standards to guide us in providing health care for the aged, both as individuals and as a group. It may indeed work well enough, much of the time, with individuals; for there we can gauge the extent to which wholeness and bodily integrity are being unavoidably lost and adapt our treatment accordingly. But when we are talking about the health of an entire age group, vital for policy analysis and for any discussion of the ends of medicine in general, we must ask where we are to find a model of wholeness. Are we to find it in that of the person who dies at the time of present average life expectancy, 75 years (which would have seemed wonderful two centuries ago), or that of the vital 90-year-old, who has shown us new possibilities? This is unmistakably a "value" choice, one that we cannot read out of nature or deduce from an analysis of classical ideas of health. How might such a choice best be made? Despite my reservations about the sufficiency of wholeness as a standard of health capable of helping us to determine the proper goals of medicine in the face of aging, it must surely have a place.

That place, I suggest, must be within an integrated understanding that takes account of two further considerations. The first is that of the wholeness of a human life. For it is perfectly possible, on the one hand, to imagine a person's body living on in a state of adequate wholeness well beyond a point at which that person's life seems to possess significance to him; and, on the other, to imagine a person's body losing its wholeness and dying well before the person has been able to live out a full life. The latter is ordinarily what we mean by a "premature death," but we really possess no common phrase to describe the former. Perhaps we can make better headway with my second consideration, the idea of a "natural life span" and a "tolerable death." By those notions I mean a fitting span of life followed by a death that is relatively acceptable in its timeliness within that life span. With those notions in hand, we could then combine the idea of health as wholeness of the body with that of some sense of the wholeness of a human life, working to bring the two ideas into a complementary relationship. Let me stress that I am not trying to read out of nature correct moral and social theories about aging and death. That may still be possible, but it is not a path I care to venture down here. I want instead to use the term "natural" in a different way, that of pointing to a persistent pattern of judgment in our culture and others of what it means to live out a life, one that manifests a wholeness and relative completeness. It can provide a realistic ideal and thus a plausible goal.

| Can There Be a "Natural Life Span" and a "Tolerable Death"?

THE PATTERN I WANT TO NOTE is a familiar one in most cultures, including our own: the belief that death at the end of a long and full life is not an evil, that indeed there is something fitting and orderly about it. As the historian of religion Frank E. Reynolds has noted in surveying a number of cultures: "The belief that human fulfillment should be sought through the indefinite postponement of physical death has appeared on the periphery of a variety of cultures. . . . However, throughout history, most men have adopted a very different attitude, one emphasizing a distinction between deaths that constitute a serious affront to human nature and those that do not. . . . [The] notion of cultural models of a meaningful life or life cycle immediately comes to the fore. Such models exist in every significant social group; a death that destroys the possibility of living out a relevant model is unnatural and abhorrent, whereas one that culminates or follows the realization of such a model is natural and at least minimally acceptable. Obviously, the identification of particular deaths as either natural or unnatural is often difficult and sometimes impossible, not only because there are degrees involved in the realization of cultural and personal goals, but also because in each society there are a variety of relevant models. Still, this distinction seems to have been recognized in one way or another in all types of human societies. . . . deaths that are recognized as natural assume the realization of a cultural or religious model of human fulfillment. In each case there is a common understanding that if an individual lives his life properly and fully, his death is divested of its negative meaning and its destructive power."[15]

What should we make of such a recurrent pattern? It surely points to the perennial human need to find a way of envisioning the fullness of a life and an acceptable conclusion to that life. The idea of life as a narrative that must have some sense and purpose, some significant degree of overall coherence and fitting closure, is an old one. If death is a reality, the end of our own personal time, then the course and direction of that time prior to the end must be given some meaning. The problem in our culture is to determine just what would be an appropriate model of the course of a life and a fitting death. That medicine seems to present an open-ended possibility— at least in the sense that it seems to deny, in its assault on disease, an acceptance of any cause of death as fitting or natural—creates an immediate obstacle. What should be an acceptable span of life and a tolerable death?

I will first propose a definition of a tolerable death. If we could agree on that, we would then have, in effect, the basis for a correlative idea of a natural life span and thus, perhaps, the foundation for an appropriate goal for medicine in its approach to aging. My definition of a "tolerable death" is this: the individual event of death at that stage in a life span when (a) one's life possibilities have on the whole been accomplished; (b) one's moral obligations to those for whom one has had responsibility have been discharged; and (c) one's death will not seem to others an offense to sense or sensibility, or tempt others to despair and rage at the finitude of human existence. Note the most obvious feature of this definition: it is a biographical, not a biological, definition. A "natural life span" may then be defined as one in which life's possibilities have on the whole been achieved and after which death may be understood as a sad, but nonetheless relatively acceptable event.

Each part of that definition requires some explanation. What do I mean when I say that "one's life possibilities have on the whole been accomplished"? I mean something very simple: that most of those opportunities which life affords people will have been achieved by that point. Life affords us a number of opportunities. These include work, love, the procreating and raising of a family, life with others, the pursuit of moral and other ideals, the experience of beauty, travel, and knowledge, among others. By old age—and here I mean even by the age of 65—most of us will have had a chance to experience those goods; and will certainly experience them by our late 70s or early 80s. It is not that life will cease, after those ages, to offer us some new opportunities; we might do something we have never done before but always sought to do. Nor is it that life will necessarily cease to offer us opportunities to continue experiencing its earlier benefits. Ordinarily it will not. But what we have accomplished by old age is the having of the opportunities themselves, and to some relatively full degree. Many people, sadly, fail to have all the opportunities they might have: they may never have found love, may not have had the income to travel, may not have gained much knowledge through lack of education, and so on. More old age is not likely to make up for those deficiencies, however; the pattern of such lives, including their deprivations, is not likely to change significantly in old age, much less open up radically new opportunities hitherto missing.

Note that my definition includes the phrase "on the whole" in referring to life's possibilities. Little imagination is required to find an exception to any of my generalizations about old age. There are people who take up jogging at 75 and compete in marathons at 80, just as there are the Grandma Moses phenomena who discover a whole new set of interests and talents in their later years. My mother took up painting in her early 70s, by 80 was selling her pictures, and continued until she died at 86. They are the exceptions. More common is the experience of not having completed all the things one would like to do. For the lifelong reader there will still be many old books not read, and a constant stream of new books to be read. For the painter, there will be an infinite number of further possibilities, as there will be for one who enjoys investing in the stock market, understanding nature, watching scientific and other knowledge being discovered, growing a garden, observing the sunset, enjoying music, and taking walks. In that sense, however, life's possibilities will never be exhausted; death at *any* time, at age 90, or 100, or 110, will frustrate those further possibilities, which are endless and likely never to be satisfied for one who has remained lively and inquiring. Yet even if we will lose such possibilities by death in old age, we will *on the whole* already have had ample time to know the pleasures of such things. That is what is most important, not that we have been unable to do everything conceivably possible, which would in any case be impossible. No amount of time would make it possible to do everything possible. The biblical idea of a full life as about three score and ten years must have had behind it a perception of that kind rather than a purely biological observation.

The greatest sadness of death at any age, including old age, is that of the definitive break it brings to love and human relationships. The steady loss of one's oldest and dearest friends is among the greatest sorrows of old age. There is nothing that medicine can do about that. More time may be of some help, but no matter how long someone lives, the grief that death brings will still be as sharp as ever. If one lives until old age, one will have had the opportunity to love and join oneself with others; 65 or 75 or 80 years is sufficient time to do that, and death at 100 or 110 or 120 will still be too soon to see our lives together come to an end.

There is perhaps one circumstance of contemporary old age that is different in some important respects from what was earlier the case. Now that subsidized retirement is possible (something that did not exist at all as a category of life until recent decades), there will be many people who, having worked hard all their lives, can have an extended time of leisure and the savoring of pleasures and experiences earlier denied them. This will be particularly true of those who were forced to endure unpleasant and unsatisfying jobs or arduous domestic duties. Retirement opens up for them the possibility of a way of life that is genuinely different and offers new opportunities (even that of simply fishing every day, or taking a walk without having to punch a time clock). There is a certain irony to be noted here, however: an increasing number of those old enough to retire are finding that they must care for their elderly parents. The same medicine and good health that have kept them alive to enjoy their retirements also keep alive their still more elderly parents, who now (especially those over 85) are likely to have some chronic illness, to be increasingly frail, and to have a greater-than-ever need for help from their children. Yet even if that does not happen, one can still ask whether the best compensation for boring and unsatisfactory jobs, or overburdened younger years, is an extended retirement. For one thing, more people are going to be forced to work into their late 60s or early 70s because of new economic pressures and Social Security disincentives against retirement. For another, it would be a much more satisfying long-term solution to seek improvement of the conditions of work in younger years than to depend upon retirement to make up the earlier deficits. Not everyone will live out a long retirement, by any means; illness may mar some or many of those years, and it is not, in any case, obvious why medicine should be called in to give what an earlier life could not.

My intention here has not been to pretend that death in old age is some unmitigated good for the person who dies. It is a loss, and the most ultimate kind of human loss. I only want to establish the plausibility of thinking that if death must come at all, death in old age after a full and—on the whole—complete life is as acceptable as death is ever likely to be for human beings. Medicine will provide only small, incremental benefits to those lives it extends beyond the 70s and early 80s; and its failure to provide those benefits would not constitute a failure on its part. If it can help us to achieve those later years, it will have given us sufficient time to experience most, if not all, of the opportunities of living a life.

The second element of my definition of a tolerable death—our obligations to others—also requires examination. When I speak of having discharged one's moral obligations, I have in mind primarily family obligations, particularly to one's children. Obligations to children are very special and inescapable. The death of parents at a time when children are still wholly dependent upon them is easily and rightly seen as particularly sad and wrong, and that is so even if others can step in and assume the parental role. It is a premature death not only biologically, but parentally and socially. Yet if the children are grown, and have achieved a self-supporting and self-directing status, it is then fair to say that the parents no longer have special obligations toward them. They have done their work in bringing their children to independence and maturity. We may be sad when an elderly person with grown children dies; but we are rarely sad (save in very special cases) because of any feeling that the children still *need* the parents as parents, even though out of affection they may miss them.

Of course there are other kinds of duties as well. Wives and husbands, by virtue of their marriage, take on mutual obligations. An ideal of many, if not most, marriages is that the spouses will so prepare themselves that the death of one will not mean the ruination or impoverishment of the other. A premature death can then be seen as one in which, for lack of time, a spouse has not been able to provide the basis for at least the material security of the survivor. But if that has been accomplished, or one lives in a sensible society that does not allow the death of a spouse to undercut all future social security of the survivor, it can be said that spouses have discharged their obligations to each other. This is by no means to deny that the survivor may be severely and permanently grieved by the death of the other. But that possibility does not seem to me sufficient to call the death wrong or untimely, though it is surely sad and wrenching, as ever it must be regardless of age.

There is still another set of obligations. What about the situation in which a person has voluntarily undertaken the duty to bear the burdens of others or to work in behalf of their improved welfare; to be a doctor, or teacher, or social worker? A premature death would, in that context, be one in which death occurred before the chosen obligations could be discharged. There are a number of difficulties in evaluating that kind of situation, however. Though a person may undertake voluntary obligations, it is not evident that an inability to discharge them can be seen as an evil. Surely there is deprivation for those who would have benefited, but others can take up their duties and continue the good work. Perhaps there is also some pain of loss on the part of those whose sense of obligation was thwarted. Yet since the obligation was voluntary, it can not easily be claimed that its beneficiaries had any right to it; the death of their benefactor cannot be counted as an injustice. Some voluntary obligations can be seen as finite and time-limited, others as open-ended and infinite. It is one thing to take responsibility for the welfare of an individual orphan and quite another to take responsibility for all orphans. More time may help in the first instance, but (assuming one can talk sensibly at all about voluntarily undertaking an obligation toward the welfare of all orphans) no amount of time is likely to make possible achievement of the second goal, if for no other reason than that more children destined to become orphans will continually be born. It is reasonable to want to help the orphans born in one's lifetime. Is it equally reasonable to feel responsible for the neglected and abandoned children in all of future history?

The third aspect of my definition—that a given death will not seem to others an offense to sense or sensibility, or elicit feelings of rage and despair at human existence—brings us to some fundamental problems about death itself. From all I can gather, the death of an elderly person who has lived a rich and full life is not, in any society, accounted an evil, as if symptomatic of a deranged and cruel universe. It may well be, of course, that mankind has simply been led to rationalize that kind of death; since it cannot be helped, it may as well be accepted. There is no way to determine if that is the case. Nor is there any way to determine if, as many (though not all) elderly testify, their proclaimed readiness to die is rationalization either. One can only point out the social fact that neither in the eyes of others nor in those of the elderly is death seen as an evil, even though it will be understood as a loss. The main reason normally given in both cases is that the elderly have lived a full life, have done what they could, and thus are not victims of the malevolence of the forces either of divinity or of nature. This seems especially true if they have, in their own eyes and those of others, completed their life's work and discharged their moral obligations to others. It is not as if life had ceased to have a purpose because of that, but instead that its *main* purposes have been achieved—both self-realization and assistance to others in their self-realization. "It is neither aging nor death itself that is objectionable," Timothy F. Murphy has written. "It is unkind aging. It is untoward death."[16]

That point may be underscored by thinking of the death of an elderly person not at the time of death or immediately thereafter, but in very distant retrospect. I can speak only from limited experience here, but I have never heard anyone remember with bitterness, or sharp regret, the death of an elderly person who lived a full and long life, but whose death occurred twenty, thirty, or forty years ago. I do not now feel sad that my paternal grandmother, who died in her early 80s some forty years ago, is dead, nor do I know of any of her own children—my father, uncles, and aunts (who were, of course, much closer to her than I was)—who remained sad for long that she was no longer alive. That most of them are now themselves dead, and their lingering sadness, if any, is buried along with them, only adds to the difficulty of imagining her death as an evil—for surely if an event had been an evil, as distinguished from an occasion for sadness, it should be possible to look back and identify just what makes it an evil even *now* (as can readily be done, for example, with the death of Anne Frank).

I would add a final stipulation about a tolerable death: that it not be marked by unbearable and degrading pain. That possibility is a major reason to make the relief of suffering a primary goal in caring for the elderly. Pain, whether physical or psychological, can destroy personality, the sense of self, and the ability to relate to others. It separates a person not only from himself but from others as well. Without attempting to develop the case in any detail, I will note that it is simply impossible that a death amidst pain or great psychological suffering could be seen by either the victim or those around him as in any sense acceptable or fitting. It is a burden in itself and impedes the realization of other goals. There was wisdom in the old idea that one should, in one's dying, be able to prepare for death and take one's leave from others in an alert way. The coming of death is a time to reflect upon the course of one's life, to heal old rifts with others if possible, to put aside the pettiness that too often marks our daily life and to consider, in the company of others, what is important and abiding. Just how often life ends in that way I have no idea, but it has happened enough in my own experience and has been reported to me enough by others that I take it to be a realistic ideal (though requiring a bit of luck perhaps, and probably some character as well). To the extent that medicine can help bring about the physical conditions necessary to make that kind of death possible, to that extent it makes a vital contribution to the wholeness of life, even if it can do no more for the wholeness of the body.

The obvious premise behind my definition of a tolerable death and a natural life span is that such a death after such a life is not an evil, even though it may well be an occasion for sadness. It is necessary to specify what I mean by evil, which I construe to be either moral or metaphysical. Death could not, at the end of a long and full life, be called a moral evil in the narrow sense of the term;

that is, in the sense that rights have been violated, a social injustice done, or clear duties defaulted. No person or persons, that is, have done wrong to the one who dies; it is the decline of the body that brings about death. Yet that is not the only sense of the term evil, which admits of other and broader manifestations. The milder form would stress the loss occasioned by meaningful potentialities forgone, that "what might have been" which can engender an acute feeling of loss at the ending of a life. The other, harsher sense of evil places the emphasis upon the absurdity and irrationality of life itself, whereby nature or fate or some other implacable and uncontrollable power victimizes hapless humans, forcing them to be born and to die in a world not of their choosing and then inflicts great harm upon them. One might call that metaphysical, as distinguished from moral, evil. That is the meaning of evil which most concerns me here; but let me look first at the milder (though still pungent) version, because it is often invoked by those who would like to see a healthy old age extended as long as possible.

The eminent gerontologists Matilda and John Riley have nicely sketched the possibilities of longer lives: "It is clear that increased longevity: (1) prolongs the opportunity for accumulating social, psychological, and biological experiences; (2) maximizes a person's opportunities to complete or to change the role assignments of early and middle life—for example, to change jobs, marriage partners, or educational plans, and to take on new roles in the later years; (3) prolongs a person's relationships to others—to spouse, parents, offspring, friends—whose lives are also extended; and (4) increases the potential structural complexity of a person's social networks—for example, of kinship, friendship, community—as all members survive longer. All these consequences of longevity mean that people now have unprecedented opportunity to accumulate experience, to exercise new and expanded options, to respond to social change, and to influence it."[7]

That is an attractive view of life, to be sure, but some doubts are in order: the other side of the ledger should be examined also. The experience that is prolonged can be misery as well as pleasure, the changing of marriage partners can leave an abandoned partner to years of loneliness, unfriendly relationships can last as well as pleasant ones, and the complexity of our networks might be a burden rather than a liberation. Chronic illness can and does weigh down the lives of many elderly. There are, after all, large numbers of people in a chronic vegetative state, or suffering from Alzheimer's disease, or permanently disabled by arthritis or dementia or stroke—people, for the most part elderly, who would not be alive at all but for the ability of medicine to extend their lives. That said, I am ready enough to grant the Rileys their point. A longer life may bring many benefits and delights for many people. But it is not evident that a failure to have such years is a self-evident *evil*; it may at worst be simply a regrettable loss.

There is also another consideration. The possibility of and the desire for the unfolding of new experiences in old age logically mean that death at no point could ever be acceptable; there would *always* be further possibilities. An unsettling result then emerges: if death must and will come at some point, then the forgoing of new or continuing possibilities of life in any one year is not necessarily worse than in any other year, especially if one would see the same range of infinite opportunities forgone in the later as in the earlier year. I note this as a paradox of death after a long life: there would always be the possibility of further benefits, pleasures, achievements, and self-realizations. Death at any time then becomes equally unacceptable—or equally acceptable. The real and ultimate problem here is that of death itself and what we are to make of it.

An immediate ambiguity presents itself. Is the real goal of medicine an indefinite extension of life—what has been called "prolongevity"—or simply a reasonably satisfactory success in coping with the problems of old age?[18] The evidence on that point is unclear, but my guess is that by its unstinting effort to conquer the causes of death, its implicit agenda is a kind of prolongevity. There is, one must suppose, at least a logical difference between seeking an indefinite extension of life and more modestly seeking only to add another twenty or thirty years. In practice, though, it may make little difference what the long-term hope is. Even the more modest goal raises many of the same problems as the search for bodily immortality. We would, in either case, do well to consider some thoughtful words of Hans Jonas on the social function of death: "the wisdom [of] the harsh dispensation [is] that it grants us the eternally renewed promise of freshness, immediacy, and eagerness of youth. . . . There is no substitute for this in the greater accumulation of prolonged experience: it can never recapture the unique privilege of seeing the world for the first time with new eyes; never relive the wonder which, according to Plato, is the beginning of philosophy. . . .This ever renewed beginning, which is only to be had at the price of ever repeated ending, may well be mankind's hope, its safeguard against lapsing into boredom and routine, its chance of retaining the spontaneity of life. . . . Perhaps a nonnegotiable limit to our expected time is necessary for each of us as the incentive to number our days and make them count."[19]

Leon Kass touches on a related point in calling our attention to a deep yet forever frustrated aspect of our human nature. "The human soul," he writes, "yearns for, longs for, aspires to some condition, some state, some goal toward which our earthly activities are directed but [which] cannot be attained during earthly life. . . . Our distress with mortality is the derivative manifestation of the conflict between the transcendent longings of the soul and the all-too-finite powers and fleshly concerns of the body."[20] Kass here draws upon many classical sources for his analysis, the Greek philosophers as well as biblical religion. Yet anyone who has reflected upon his or her own life, and particularly on the fleetingness of pleasure and deep satisfactions, can well understand what those ancients were striving to grasp. It is not simply that our mortality as a whole makes it difficult for us to hold on to the pleasures of life; the very limited nature of those pleasures even at their very best—frustratingly bittersweet and evanescent—leads us to long for more. What is that "more"? Whatever it is, a mere extension of life will not satisfy those deeper longings of the spirit; time cannot provide them. Instead, "Once we acknowledge and accept our finitude, we can concern ourselves with living well, and care first and most for the *well-being* of our souls, and not so much for their mere existence. . . . to covet a prolonged life span for ourselves is both a sign and a cause of our failure to open ourselves to . . . any higher . . . purpose."[21]

I believe Kass is right in what he discerns; but there is also another side to the story. Whatever deeper and wider reasons, whether religious or biological, we might find to support the value of death, it is also part of our natural endowment that we want to live and not to die. It is a sign of our greatest vitality, a symbol of our joy in the riches of existence, a mark of our striving to find that which makes us most human. Should this not count as a contradiction to the kind of arguments Kass advances? One possible response is that very old age itself resolves the contradiction by diminishing the will to live. Many elderly people report the loss of a desire for more life, find themselves weary of the effort to cope with social change, or the loss of their friends, and strongly affirm their willingness to accept death. Yet that is by no means the case with all old persons, many of whom struggle against their death until the very end. The impact of weakness and debility on those who say they are ready to give up on life is often hard to gauge. If they felt better and stronger, they might well be prepared to live on.

The exact significance, in short, of statements by the old of their willingness to die is not obvious in its import. If any final resolution is to be found, it is more likely to come through some sense of a transcendent value or redeeming outcome in death. For many religious believers, the possibility of immortality offers such a hope. Even those who do not share that belief may find significance in the passing of the generations, seeing in death, with Leon Kass, a biological value to younger generations of sufficient power to afford at least some amelioration of the violence that death, and the thought of death, does to the sense of individuality and the will to live. Even so, it is hard to see how anyone who lives a decent life, one unburdened by serious illness or emotional problems and blessed with the love and support of others, would gladly take leave of life. It is precious. At best we can find some abstract purpose in death, even if no coherent or comforting resolution is ultimately possible. However we may understand those matters, one point should be evident: a longer and healthier old age will not provide the ultimate answer to death or remove its sting.

| Ends of Aging/Ends of Medicine

IT IS TIME TO FILL OUT the remainder of my argument. I have tried to make plausible the claim that the appropriate goal of medicine as it confronts aging is not the extension of life as such, but the achievement of a full and natural life span. As it confronts aging, medicine should have as its specific goals averting premature death, understood as death before the fulfillment of a natural life span, and the relief of suffering. It should pursue those goals in order that the elderly can finish out their years with a conviction that their lives have meaning and significance, with as little suffering as possible, with as much vigor as possible in contributing to the welfare of the young and the community of which they are a part. By vigor I do not exclusively mean active, physical vigor. Beyond some point of physical decline and with the approach of death, there may be little of that left. I take it also to be vigor of a no less valuable kind, to present to the young a model of what it means to decline gracefully, to relinquish roles and visibility, and to reflect on the way death closes out a life. Even that latter kind of vigor, which may be manifest only as a struggle for some kind of tranquillity, may well require the ministrations of medicine. Medicine cannot bring happiness, but it can help provide the physical substrate of a tolerable aging and death. Those in the process of aging, or already aged, should ask of medicine not a longer life, but help in maintaining a life that can complete its work as close to the time of death as possible. More needs to be said, however, about the relief of suffering and maintenance of function.

The cure of disease and the relief of suffering, each representing a threat to human wholeness, have long been accepted as appropriate goals of medicine. Disease destroys the wholeness and integrity of the body, and pain and suffering can destroy the wholeness of the person. While medicine is well honed to combat pain, suffering is a more complex category, which may but does not necessarily involve the presence of pain. It is a particularly important problem in caring for the aged. Aging portends the dissolution of more than the body. "Suffering," Eric Cassell has written, "occurs when an impending destruction of the person is perceived; it continues until the threat of disintegration has passed or until the integrity of the person can be restored in some other manner."[22] In the case of the aging, the threat will not pass. How can it be softened? Fear of the future, an acute source of suffering, will be an element in aging, particularly toward the end. There is no future, and that may be the hardest thing to accept. How is that to be tolerated? Cassell offers some helpful insights: "Meaning and transcendence offer two . . . ways by which the suffering associated with destruction of a part of personhood is ameliorated. Assigning a meaning to the injurious condition often reduces or even resolves the suffering associated with it. . . . Transcendence is probably the most powerful way in which one is restored to wholeness after an injury to personhood. When experienced, transcendence locates the person in a far larger landscape. The sufferer is not isolated by pain but is brought closer to a transpersonal source of meaning and to the human community that shares those meanings."[23] Cassell does not define "transcendence," but I would urge that a sense that one has lived out one's final years helping those who will remain is one important source of it.

A medicine oriented toward the relief of suffering will, in the case of the elderly, be a medicine that is concerned with the sick person, not the sickness of the person. The disease or combination of diseases that will be the actual cause of death and the source of pain can only be ameliorated, not cured; or, if it should be cured, it is understood that its place will soon be taken by another. The relief of pain may pose a special dilemma. For some at least, mental clarity in the presence of pain may be preferable to the drowsiness or stupefaction induced by pain relievers. For others, the terror of pain induced by some conditions may lead them in a different direction, such as heavy doses of morphine. In caring for a person who is trying to find meaning in a life coming to an end, different kinds of preference should be respected; it is the person as a whole who is the subject of treatment. But so far as possible, the goal of the physician should be to reduce the physical obstacles that impede the search for the meaning and transcendence which can make the suffering bearable. The further extension of life would then become a secondary goal, if a goal at all. The point is that life has now come to an end, and there is only one question of importance: what does a person need to secure at its closing the greatest possible integrity? Since more life as such is rarely the answer to that problem, then a high goal of a medicine for the aged will be the management of suffering. That this kind of medical care requires skills and understanding which go well beyond technical knowledge need not be stressed. That physicians and other health-care workers must here be prepared to spend time in talking with the elderly, and giving of themselves to them, is a prime duty.

What would a medicine be like that was oriented toward the relief of suffering rather than the deliberate extension of life? We do not yet have a clear answer to that question readily at hand, so longstanding, central, and persistent has been the struggle against death as a part of the self-conception of medicine. But the hospice movement is providing us with much helpful evidence. It knows how to distinguish between the relief of suffering and the extension of life. "The relief of suffering" means at least the control of pain and an active effort to promote physical functioning, mental alertness, and emotional stability. Medicine cannot by itself supply meaning and significance to the late years. That can be achieved only by the elderly person and by the larger society. But a life marked by pain, depression, and radical loss of physical function cannot be a life well positioned to seek a larger good. Those inflictions have a devastating way of turning one in upon oneself, of blotting out all other possibilities, and of inducing despair. A medicine that can relieve a heavy weight of that kind will be a splendid medicine. But can medical practice, as a general rule, play that role?

The most disturbing impediment has been well characterized by an article whose title tells its story: "Longer Life but Worsening Health? Trends in Health and Mortality of Middle-Aged and Older Persons."[24] This study is but one of a number that have tried to gauge the impact of longer life on the health of the old and on the need for health resources. Among its author's findings are increased restriction of activity through bed disability, a sharp increase in total restriction of activity, a steady growth in the percentage of those limited in primary (job, housework) and secondary activities, and a rise in the prevalence and impact of both lethal chronic diseases (cancer, stroke) and of those which do not kill but limit activity (arthritis, sinusitis). In one respect, trends of this kind are a backhanded kind of compliment to acute-care medicine and generally improved health information: more people are being saved from death, and more people are aware of, and reporting, chronic illness.

But there is no doubt also that this is a phenomenon closely associated with an aging population, and one that directly calls into question the way medicine is progressing. Such occurrences are surely "the failures of success."[25] A medicine prone to trade acute for chronic illness has a problem of its self-conception on its hands. But chronic illness is an inevitable outcome in a medicine that has among its patients an increasingly larger proportion of the elderly and that becomes steadily more skilled at saving those elderly people from death.[26]

James Fries provoked considerable attention in the early 1980s by his writings on "The Compression of Morbidity." His was the interesting prediction that medicine in the future would not see a great increase in the number of the elderly, but that chronic disease would decrease along with the need for medical care, and that there would be a drop in the average period of decreased vigor prior to death. At the heart of these projections was the concept of compressed morbidity and senescence followed by a quick death—a "squaring of the curve," as it came to be called, of old age and death.[27] Since in Fries's view the length of human life is fixed, an average life span would be about 85 years; we would live healthy, alert lives until that age, and then experience a quick death. Whether that is a feasible goal medically is far less clear, and the trend to date is not encouraging. There is little evidence of a decline in morbidity and disability among the very old, and an increasing number of people are living well beyond 85.[28] Even so—and a far longer period of time will be needed to evaluate its feasibility—the "compression of morbidity" rather than the extension of life is a goal consistent with what I have been arguing for here. An improvement of *active* life expectancy, not life expectancy in itself, would be medicine's purpose.[29] As Fries and many others have indicated, moreover, there are a number of ways in which that goal can be pursued, particularly by preventive medicine and good health habits from an early age.[30] In short, even if Fries is wrong in his belief that morbidity can be compressed, and that there is a set life expectancy, he may be right in his ideals. We are not required to continue chasing an indefinite life extension. We can settle for the achievement of a limited, natural life span. That would be sufficient, and would allow the possibility of concentrating on improving the quality of life prior to the end of that life span.

Unlike the goal of extending life, that of seeking to improve the quality of life of the elderly points to an important set of additional considerations which should be part of medicine's self-reflection. How should the good that is health, a primary good certainly, be understood in the constellation of other human goods? These include education, culture, economic prosperity, national defense, scientific research outside the health arena, and so on. Health itself, we sometimes need reminding, is a means and not an end. We can do nothing with good health itself; it makes other human goods possible. But we need to know what those goods are and how they are to be balanced against the value of health. A goal of the extension of life combined with an insatiable desire for improvement in health—a longer and simultaneously better life for the elderly—is a recipe for monomania and bottomless spending. It fails to put health in its proper place, fails to accept aging and death as part of the human condition, and fails to present to younger generations a model of wise stewardship. A goal of aging that stresses the needs of the future generations, not only those of the old, and a goal of medicine that stresses the avoidance of premature death and the relief of suffering would together provide an alternative to our present situation.

4 | What Do the Young Owe the Old?

THE PRIMARY ASPIRATION of the aged, I have proposed, should be to advance not their own welfare but that of the young and the generations to come. They are stewards of the world they helped fashion in earlier years and must now turn over to others. That ideal could be attractive to the elderly only as part of a view of medicine and aging which accepts limits to the enterprise of conquering disease and forestalling death, and which therefore accepts limits to their own lives. This is, admittedly, to ask a great deal of the elderly, conditioned as we all are to expect a relentless conquest of nature for our well-being, and desirous of a healthy and long life. If the elderly are, moreover, to be asked to direct themselves to younger generations, what assurance can they have that they will not be neglected, abused, or exploited in the process?

That assurance must be promoted, and can be achieved only by the flourishing of social values, practices, and institutions which prize the elderly and seek to improve their welfare. But is it possible to respect their dignity, to fully acknowledge their contributions and accomplishments, and yet still—at the same time—contemplate a limit to some forms of health care? I believe it both possible and necessary; but much will depend upon the way in which we ground and proclaim the respect due the elderly and then embody it in our daily practices and institutional arrangements. That the old have powerful obligations toward the young in no way relieves the latter of their own distinctive duties toward the old. On the contrary, the sacrifices to be asked of the old on behalf of the young will require a fresh commitment of the young to the old. How should we understand that commitment and the duties it carries with it?

Let us start at the most basic levels. The elderly are members of families, and thus part of familial and intimately personal networks of moral obligation. They are also members of an age group that enters into relationships with other, younger age groups, both through the impersonal medium of welfare and medical-care programs and through more informal social, civic, and professional interactions. The young can minimally (if hardly adequately) discharge their formal social obligations to the elderly merely by paying taxes to support entitlement programs for them. That straitened construal of duty is, however, all too readily compatible with treating the elderly on a personal level in a demeaning or abusive way.[1] Young family members can similarly take loving care of their own elderly parents or relatives while systematically ignoring the legitimate needs of other elderly people. To discharge well our familial obligations to our own elderly relatives is not automatically to discharge our broader social obligations to the elderly as an age group. The two are equally important in any rounded view of what the young owe the old.

Yet if there are both familial and general duties toward the old, we must find the proper boundaries between them. We need to have some sense of what we can legitimately, in the name of filial obligation, ask and expect of families in the care of their own elderly, and what the reasonable limits to such expectations ought to be. Since we will look reasonably to government to do what families cannot or should not be called upon to do, we need no less to know where the duties and limits to help from that quarter can be found. While I will discuss in detail family roles and obligations, a caution is in order at the outset. By no means do all elderly persons have families to which they can turn for help, either because their nearest kin are no longer alive, or because their families are unable or unwilling to provide adequate care and affection. Realism must therefore temper any general discussion of the role of families. In some cases, the family can be looked to for help; in others, that will simply be impossible and the larger society will be the only resource available.

| Children and Elderly Parents: Filial Obligations

IN THE SPRING OF 1983 the Reagan Administration announced that states could as part of the Medicaid program legally require children to contribute to the support of their elderly parents. At that time a number of states were considering or enacting just such laws, whose obvious intent was to reduce state support of the elderly. The Administration, one spokesman said, was not proposing anything inherently new. It was simply responding to a state request for clarification of the existing Medicaid law, and wanted only to say that state statutes enforcing family-responsibility laws were not in conflict with federal policy.[2] Whether that response was ingenuous or contrived is not clear. As it turned out, the Administration backed down, seeing immediately that its proposal lacked public support and was an initiative whose time had not yet come. While a number of states flirted for a time with new family-responsibility policies, only a few (Virginia, Idaho, and Mississippi, for example) actually adopted them, and even fewer seem to have enforced them.

The Administration's initiative was, nonetheless, an important social and policy event. Finding acceptable ways to induce children to provide care for their aged parents will, in the face of rising costs, exert a growing attraction. The pressures and incentives in that direction are powerful, displaying a mix of financial, ideological, and charitable motives. Yet if children are going to be asked to take on greater burdens, then some fundamental questions need to be asked. What kind of moral obligation do children have toward the welfare of their elderly parents? What are the limits of that obligation? Even if children do have some significant duties to parents, is it still legitimate to ask the state to take over much of the direct financial burden of care?

We might begin answering those questions by noting first what children actually do for their parents. Gerontologists take great pleasure in demolishing what they tell us are two prevalent myths: that the caring family has disappeared and that the elderly are isolated from their children. There has indeed been a decline in the proportion of elderly who live with their children or other relatives, from three-fifths in 1960 to one-third in 1980, and to an estimated one-sixth at present.[3] There has been an equally sharp drop—down to 1 percent—in the number of elderly who depend upon their children for financial support.[4] Yet it seems still to be true, as Ethel Shanas has noted, that "most old people live close to at least one of their children and see at least one child often. Most old people see their siblings and relatives often, and old people, whether bedfast or housebound because of ill health, are twice as likely to be living at home as to be residents in an institution."[5] Between 60 and 80 percent of all disabled or impaired persons receive significant family help.[6]

Yet there have been changes in both practices and attitudes. The proportion of young and old who believe that children should be financially responsible for their elderly parents has shifted downward (from about 50 percent in the mid-1950s to 10 percent in the mid-1970s), and a simultaneous reduction in actual financial assistance has occurred.[7] This need not be taken as an indication of a diminished sense of filial responsibility. The advent of Social Security and the otherwise increasing financial strength of the elderly are both important social variables which have reduced financial pressure on children to support parents. Other social changes could eventually alter the parent-child bond. The increasing number of single parents, the complicated family relationships resulting from a high divorce rate, small families, and families in which both spouses work have together created the possibility of a reduced sense of obligation in the future.[8] Though such a possibility has yet clearly to materialize, some hints of it are in the air. In his 1981 book *New Rules*, Daniel Yankelovich, summarizing public-opinion surveys, wrote that "one of the most far-reaching changes in [moral] norms relates to what parents believe they owe their children and what their children owe them. Nowhere are the changes in the unwritten social contract more significant or agonizing. The overall pattern is clear: today's parents expect to make fewer sacrifices for their children than in the past, but they also demand less from their offspring in the form of future obligations than their parents demanded of them. . . . Sixty-seven percent [of Americans surveyed] believe that 'children do not have an obligation to their parents regardless of what their parents have done for them.' "9

To what extent this shift, assuming it is real, will lead to a change in the behavior and attitudes noted earlier remains to be seen. According to other available data and most commentators, children and families strongly remain the principal source of emotional support and companionship for the elderly.10 There is at the same time a pronounced distaste on the part of both children and parents for burdening children with financial obligations toward their parents.11 Contemporary life, it seems widely assumed, requires a different moral standard. No doubt part of the reason for this assumption is the longer life span of the elderly, the much higher cost of caring for them, and the greater demands on families in caring for their own children.

That we should as a society respect and care for the elderly is a proposition that, if stated vaguely enough, would command widespread agreement. A community that did not care for its elderly would not be a moral community. Yet if we asked people precisely *why* we should feel this way, we would probably get a wide range of answers. There are, it turns out, many espoused reasons for concern about the elderly, but they are not all of a kind: their dependency, their frailty, their maturity, their wisdom, for instance. But not all of the elderly are dependent, frail, mature, or wise. Nor is it self-evident why we should respect the elderly as a group simply because they are old, or as individual old people simply because of their age.

While piety toward the elderly was accounted a high virtue in classical Greek and Roman societies, and has had its place in the Western religions (though not so high a one, and more focused on filial obligation), its precise historical basis is not clear. That the aged pass on to the young the values and traditions of a culture was one reason. Closely related was the idea that the elderly possess wisdom, which is gained only from living, and suffering, a long and reflective life. They know, or should know, things that the young cannot yet know but need to know. The principle of reciprocity— that the young owe a debt to the old, just as one day their children will owe a debt to them—appears also to be a persistent, if often tacit, conviction in most societies. The generations are understood to be inextricably linked with each other, and respect for the elderly is an abiding and central part of that bond.[12]

At the root of that system of reciprocity, providing its model instance, is the parent–child bond. The biblical injunction to "Honor thy father and thy mother" expresses that value. But each generation has had to make its own sense of that command. It neither tells us in what "honor" consists nor how far filial obligation should be carried. As a piece of practical advice, however, it once made considerable sense. In most traditional and agricultural societies, parents had considerable power over the lives of their offspring. Children who did not honor their parents, especially their fathers, risked not only immediate privation, but also the loss of the one inheritance that would allow them adequately to raise and support their own families, land they could call their own.[13] The advent of industrialization brought the beginning of some radical changes, among them a growing place for government in taking on problems that could no longer be left to the family. It also reduced the coercive power of parents over their children, setting in motion a trend toward the independence of both parents and children that has been the mark of contemporary life. Yet the persistence of the biological and emotional bonds between children and parents has provided the opportunistic occasion for government, now feeling overwhelmed in its welfare role, to see the possibility of reducing its own burdens.

Some twenty-six states at present have statutes that can require children to provide financial support for needy parents. Though erratically administered, difficult to implement, and of doubtful financial value, they remain as testimony to periodic efforts dating back to the early seventeenth century to shift from the public to the private sphere the care of poverty-stricken elderly. While such laws had no precedent in either common law or medieval law, they came into being in England with the Elizabethan Poor Law of 1601, which represented a culmination of at least three centuries of efforts to cope with the problem of the poor in general. The Poor Law did not concentrate on the children of the elderly, but extended the network of potential support to include the fathers and mothers, and the grandfathers and grandmothers, of the poor. The family, as a unit, was to be responsible for poverty-stricken kinfolk.

When such laws passed over into the American scene during the seventeenth and eighteenth centuries, their focus was on the responsibility of children toward their elderly parents, though a few states have retained the wider scope.[14] Blackstone's famous *Commentaries* succinctly states the moral basis of such a responsibility: "The duties of children to their parents arise from a principle of natural justice and retribution. For to those who gave us existence we naturally owe subjection and obedience during our minority, and honor and reverence ever after; they who protected the weakness of our infancy are entitled to our protection in the infirmity of their age; they who by sustenance and education have enabled their offspring to prosper ought in return to be supported by that offspring in case they stand in need of assistance."[15] The American state laws were little invoked during the eighteenth and nineteenth centuries, but they have been increasingly turned to during the twentieth century, particularly in the aftermath of the Depression and World War II.

While there is broad historical agreement that the primary purpose of the filial-obligation laws was to protect the public from the burden of caring for the poor, including the elderly, the laws were buttressed by a variety of moral assumptions.[16] Martin R. Levy and Sara W. Gross have identified three moral premises that underlie the American laws and have developed some cogent criticisms of them. The first is simple reciprocity: "the duty of a child to support his parents is a mirror-image of the parents' responsibility to support a child."[17] They point out the doubtful logic of that position. In procreation, parents not only bring a child into the world, but by the same action undertake the moral obligation of sustaining that child, whose existence is entirely dependent upon the parents. The relationship of the child to the parent is different. "The child has not acted to bring about the life of the parent. While the father assumes the voluntary status of fatherhood, the child assumes no duty by having been born."[18] While Levy and Gross do not deny that there can be a moral bond of love and affection, "moral duty and gratitude, or lofty ideals, cannot be used as a justification for the taking of property"; that is, parents cannot lay claim to the goods or income of their children on the basis of those ideals.[19]

The second general moral premise turns on what they call "the relational interest of family status."[20] They mean by that phrase that the simple fact of a family relationship—creating a special tie between parent and child, both biological and social—may itself engender a demand made upon children to support their elderly parents. Yet they point out that the relational interest is both too broad and too narrow to serve as a reasonable criterion for determining the duty of children to provide support. "It is too broad in . . . that not all children love and revere their parents. The status of a child confers no special emotional tie in and of itself."[21] It is too narrow in that if emotional commitment is the standard, then a child would logically be bound to support everyone to whom he or she is tied by emotional commitment, whether family member or not.[22]

The analogy of a contract provides the third moral premise. Since the child was at one time supported by the parent, does not that create an implicit contract requiring that the child in turn support the parent when that becomes necessary? Not necessarily. No direct contract is negotiated between parent and child when the child is procreated, and any analogy must thus be based on an implied or quasi-contract. But the analogy of an implied contract does not work: the two parties necessary to the making of a contract did not exist simultaneously. A common standard in the law, moreover, is that neither the carrying out of a duty nor the promise of rendering a performance already required by duty is a sufficient condition of a return promise—that is, an obligation to do likewise.[23]

The argument that the benefits bestowed by parents upon children automatically entail a duty of the children in return to aid parents can, then, be effectively neutralized. Yet a relatively narrow focus on strict obligation does not exhaust the issue. Are we to hold, for instance, that obligation flows in one direction only, from parent to child, and that because children were given no choice about being born, they owe nothing to their parents? That view seems too extreme. It fails to explain why in fact many children feel a powerful obligation toward their parents, and does not sufficiently plumb the moral depths of the family relationship.

The philosopher Jane English suggested an alternative approach. "The duties of grown children," she wrote, "are those of friends and result from love between them and their parents, rather than being things owed in repayment for the parents' earlier sacrifices."[24] In situations wherein one person does a favor for another, there may be an obligation to reciprocate; but parents do not do favors for their children in the same sense in which strangers or acquaintances may do them for one another. The bond that should unite parents and children is that of friendship. "Friendship ought to be characterized *by mutuality* rather than reciprocity: friends offer what they can give and accept what they need without regard for the total amount of benefits exchanged. And friends are motivated by love rather than by the prospect of repayment. Hence, talk of 'owing' is singularly out of place in friendship."[25] Thus children ought to do those things which help and benefit their parents, but the "ought" is that which follows from friendship. It resists both quantitative measurement and the stricter language of owing something in return for earlier benefits.

While English's argument has some plausibility, it is ultimately unsatisfying. Friendship can certainly exist between parent and child, but it often does not. They may come to have little in common other than their biological relationship. The nature of the friendship, moreover, that exists between parent and child can and usually will be different from the kind that exists between and among those who are unrelated. A child might credibly say that while he is not a friend of his parents', he nonetheless feels toward them respect and love. Many children actively dislike their parents, find no pleasure in their company, and yet feel they ought to help them despite those feelings. It is one more example, yet a telling one, of the way in which love and hate can be intertwined.

Another powerful candidate for the source of filial obligation is gratitude on the part of children toward their parents. Gratitude may be due not simply because the parents discharged their obligations toward their children, but because in their manner of doing so they went beyond the demands of mere duty, giving voluntarily of themselves in a way neither required nor ordinarily expected of them. No less important is the motivation of those who help us. "Duties of gratitude," Jeffrey Blustein has noted, "are owed only to those who have helped or benefited us freely, without thought of personal gain, simply out of a desire to protect or promote our well-being. The givers may hope for some return, but they do not give in expectation of it."[26] But parents ordinarily have and raise children for their own benefit and pleasure as well as that of the children. Only rarely is childbearing wholly altruistic, even if marked by self-giving of a high order.

Even so, we might readily agree with Joel Feinberg when he writes, "My benefactor once freely offered me his services when I needed them. . . . But now circumstances have arisen in which he needs help, and I am in a position to help him. Surely, I owe him my services now, and he would be entitled to resent my failure to come through."[27] A qualification is in order here: gratitude is ordinarily thought due only when, as noted above, a benefactor has gone beyond ordinary duties. In some cases, parents may have done their duty, but in such a grudging way that no gratitude seems due them. We are then brought back to the original problem: how accurately to characterize the duties of children toward parents.

The origin and nature of the parent–child bond is unique in human relationships. By the procreation of children, parents create a social unit that otherwise would not and could not exist. If children do not select their parents, neither do parents select their individual children (they choose to have *a* child, not *this* child). Even so, the family relationship is not something one can simply take or leave. It is a fundamental and unavoidable element in our social nature as human beings. That psychotherapists can spend a good deal of time untangling problems between parents and children provides at least a clue to the emotional depth engendered by the biological relationship. We can and do drift away from ordinary friendships, but parents stay in our memory and exert their influence even over distance or in the face of active hostility. Whether we like it or not, we are in some sense always one with our parents both because of the unique circumstances by which we came to know them and because of the long period of nurture when we were utterly dependent upon them. The emotional and biological bond between parent and child gives the relationship a permanent and central place in our lives, quite apart from whether that relationship turns out well or poorly. That cannot usually be said of friendship in the ordinary sense of the term; it is probably no accident that psychoanalysts seem infrequently called upon to untangle the relationships between friends.

Ferdinand Schoeman catches some of this flavor when he argues that the traditional language of morality, that of rights and obligations, does not seem to fit well in describing the bond among family members: "We *share ourselves* with those with whom we are intimate and are aware that they do the same with us. Traditional moral boundaries, which give rigid shape to the self, are transparent to this kind of sharing. This makes for nonabstract moral relationships in which talk about rights of others, respect for others, and even welfare of others is to a certain extent irrelevant."[28] Perhaps Schoeman takes things too far, but he tries to make clear that the intimacy of family relationships forces us into revealing and sharing with each other facets of ourselves that may not be revealed to others on the public stage. We see each other unfolding, creating bonds of a unique kind, matched by no other human relationship. While it is often the case that parents do not really know their own child, just as often they do, even when their perceptions differ from those of the child. Whether they understand their child or not, the fact that they shared considerable intimacy when the child was young gives them access to a self which others may never see. For their part, children have unique acess to parents, knowing a side of them which may never be revealed to others.

I am searching here with some difficulty for a way to characterize the nature of the parent–child relationship, a relationship that appears almost but not quite self-evident in its reciprocal moral claims and yet oddly elusive also. To reduce the relationship to equal mutual moral duties, rights, and obligations implies a rigor and formalism that distorts the felt actuality of the moral bond as well as going beyond what can rationally be defended. If we try to make it a matter of voluntary affection only, however, we seem to say too little. Yet we cannot, I suspect, totally dismiss the language of obligation, nor would we want to give up the ideal of mutual affection either. If the procreation and physical rearing of a child does not automatically entail reciprocal duties toward the parents when they are needy and dependent, it is certainly possible to imagine a sense of obligation arising when parents have done far more for children than would morally be required of them. My own parents, for example, did not drop me when I reached eighteen. They sacrificed a good deal to provide me with a higher education, and in fact provided financial support for my graduate education until I was thirty, topping that off by giving my wife and me a down payment on our first house. They did it out of affection, rather than duty, but I certainly felt I owed them something in return in their old age. There need not be, then, any necessary incompatibility in feeling both affection and a sense of duty. But we lack a moral phrase that catches both notions in one concept; and neither taken separately is quite right.

| The Power of Need and Dependence

ANOTHER ASPECT OF THE RELATIONSHIP between children and their elderly parents bears reflection. Much as young children will have a special dependence upon parents, as those human beings above all others who have a fateful power over their destinies, so, in dire circumstances, many elderly parents can come to depend similarly upon their children. In a world of strangers or fleeting casual acquaintances, of distant government agencies and a society beyond their control, elderly parents can see in their children their only hope for someone who ought to care for them. Neither parent nor child may want this kind of emotional dependence, and each might wish that there were an alternative. Nonetheless, while many elderly parents are able to form strong bonds of attachment with friends and neighbors, some parents may be forced to throw themselves upon their children simply because there is no other choice. Who else is likely to care?

Can that sense of utter need, if not necessarily for money then only for affection and caring, in and of itself create a moral obligation? It is surely a difficult question whether, as a general matter, a moral obligation is incurred when one human being is rendered by circumstance wholly dependent upon another. Can the dependence itself create the obligation, quite apart from any other features of the relationship? A moral claim of that kind will inevitably be controversial, if only because it is common to rest strict claims of obligation only upon implicit or explicit contracts of one kind or another—promises we have made or implicit commitments entailed by our actions (one of which may be procreation). It is difficult in the case of elderly parents plausibly to invoke such norms (short, of course, of the child's having made a voluntary, explicit promise). Still, the power of sheer dependence—whether of a newborn child upon a parent or of an elderly, dependent parent upon a child—can be potent in its experienced moral demands.[29] The fate of one or more persons rests in the hands of another. The issue, as it presents itself, may be less one of trying to discover the grounds of obligation that would require a response than one of trying to find a basis for ignoring a demand that so patently assaults the sensibilities. It is not so much "Must I?" as it is "How can I not?"

In trying to unravel the nature of the possible moral obligation, it may be helpful to speak of some specific claims or demands that might be made. Money is no longer the only, or necessarily the most important, benefit that elderly parents actually ask of their children. On a scale of moral priorities, in any case, it would be difficult persuasively to argue that persons in a middle generation have an obligation to deprive their own dependent children of necessary financial support in order to support their elderly parents. By virtue of their having procreated those children, the latter have a claim upon them which their parents cannot equal. Of course, where a surplus exists after their own children have been taken care of, the financial support of needy parents might become obligatory, particularly if there were no other available sources of support. Ordinarily, however, the principal economic duties of adults will be toward their own children rather than toward their parents.

The same cannot necessarily be said of providing either physical help or affection to their parents. While the giving of physical help and giving of affection could readily be merged, I think it is useful to distinguish between them. Physical help—such as assistance in moving, cleaning, shopping, and trips to visit friends or doctors, or supervision of home attendants—is a somewhat different contribution to the welfare of the elderly from simply talking with them. Parents of young children may not readily be able to adapt their schedules to strenuous physical demands of that kind upon their time or energy. Yet they may be able to provide affection, either by visits at times they find convenient, or through letters and telephone calls. An inability to provide some kinds of care does not exempt children from providing other forms; in fact, the available evidence suggests that what is most wanted by elderly parents is affection. It is not difficult to understand why. Isn't that what we all need? That need is intensified in the elderly. The uncertainties of old age, the recognition of growing weakness and helplessness, can above all generate the desire to believe that at least some people in the world care about one's fate and are willing empathically to share that burden which few of us would care to bear alone: a recognition that life is gradually coming to an end, that nature is depriving us of our body and our future.[30] Sensitive children will be aware of that need in their parents, and emotional support will be part of an ideal parent–child relationship.

The moral ideal of the parent–child relationship is love, nurture, and the mutual seeking of the good of the other. While the weight of the relationship will ordinarily shift according to the ages of children and their parents, mutual respect and reciprocity have been a central part of the moral standard. Yet the realities of human life can stand in the way of the realization of moral ideals; they usually do. Not all children are lovable, and not all parents give the welfare of their children their serious attention and highest priority. Many children, in turn, do not find their parents endearing and feel no special sense of duty toward them. To what extent and under what circumstances flaws and faults of that kind can be said to alter the mutual obligations is obviously an important question. Yet even when the affectional bonds between parent and child are strong, it is still by no means clear what each morally owes the other. If children should honor their elderly parents, how great a sacrifice ought that to entail?

| Imperative Duties and Impossible Demands

THAT QUESTION IS DISTURBING but unavoidable, given the trend to return to families and the home the care of the chronically ill and the frail elderly. The possibly dubious assumption behind this trend is that families will, with some modest degree of social support, be able practically to manage such care and have the moral, psychological, and spiritual strength to do so. I am not certain about that assumption, at least in the case of a frail, sick, or demented parent who may require many months or years of demanding, stressful care. That there is an obligation of children to provide time and affection, and physical help when possible, to their elderly parents is not in dispute. The limits to such support, and the proper context for claiming it, are less clear.

At its best, and even perhaps when everything is far from ideal, the care of the elderly by their children can be a mutually rewarding experience. It can join families together more tightly, allow the discovery of new depths of love and devotion, and provide many opportunities for growth and self-knowledge. But it is important not to romanticize the possibilities, however often things turn out well for many families. The care of frail or ill elderly family members can also be an occasion of oppression and hostility. The child is often trapped in a way of life and a future direction not of his or her own choice. Our secular morality (though perhaps not our religious traditions) provides few resources for living lives of unchosen obligations, those which through mischance lay upon us overwheming demands to give our life over to the succor and welfare of someone else. The idea of a return to traditional forms of support is, in that respect, both ironic and appealing. Part of the ideology behind medical and technological progress is that of liberating human life from the inexorability of bodily decay and disability and, at the same time, from the uninvited and smothering social burdens they impose on our lives. That the more advanced stages of that progress should lead us back to an embracing of just those same burdens as a way of coping with the progress is an ironic outcome.

The more appealing (and seductive) impetus behind this trend is in part the financial pressure occasioned by the growing social burden of disability among the frail elderly. An ever-growing number of the elderly are kept alive for an ever-longer period of time, but at the price of ever-extended care and rehabilitation to ensure their continuing survival and well-being. The full provision of such care by government funds or institutions promises to be insupportable. Soon there will be too many people needing too much care. What is to be done? The popular answer is to widen the scope and acceptability of family care.³¹ That promises to be a less expensive solution. A supporting motive is a widespread belief that family care as a focus of public policy can often be superior care, more kindly and sensitive, more acutely attuned to the needs of individuals, and more compatible with some significant traditional values, notably those of kinship and family integrity.

What kinds of moral and psychological resources are necessary to carry out such a policy? Even if children are willing to care for their elderly parents, where can they personally find the necessary strength, endurance, and stability to sustain their commitment and, no less important, to make moral sense of it? That is a question they will ask themselves, and if the stress is intensive and unrelieved, perhaps find no answer. How will society honor and help them, and how will it provide an honored social significance to complement and reinforce whatever individual meaning they may bring to bear? That is a question we should ask on their behalf, and perhaps we will not readily find an answer. We can moralize easily enough about keeping our promises, honoring our commitments, and respecting our contracts. But if doing so in the circumstance of extended life spans—well beyond what earlier generations knew—begins to threaten our psychological survival, our basic social freedom, our otherwise legitimate private hopes and plans, then only the best-rooted, the most cogent reasons and compelling emotions are likely to sustain us.

That goal is not easy to achieve in our society. We lack, as a people, any common coherent vision of the wellsprings of moral obligation toward the elderly in general and our elderly parents in particular. We do not have a shared understanding of the moral significance of pain and suffering, or any clear notion of how we ought to support one another's private griefs and burdens. We do not provide strong encouragement for those personal virtues which enable people to endure in the face of adversity. All of those communal deficits can come to a high intensity in the demands that vulnerable elderly parents can make upon their children. Their claim upon us can well seem, and often may well be, insupportable.

It is an old and hard moral question to know what we should make of severe demands for self-sacrifice. Most moral rules have common sense and practicality to commend them. Murder, lying, and theft ordinarily have tangibly bad consequences for those who commit such acts. Even our self-interest commands us to avoid them. Matters are otherwise when we are morally asked to give up our lives, or personal hopes, for the sake of another. Only under special circumstances can that seem to make any sense at all from the viewpoint of self-interest, even of the most benign sort. It is not for nothing that almost all Western moralities have been careful to distinguish between what we must do as a matter of duty and what we heroically might do. They all recognize that a morality designed to apply to a whole community cannot require that everyone be a saint or a model of altruism. The notion that we might as a matter of social policy burden families with the heavy duty of caring for their frail elderly ought at least to raise a flag of warning about the possibility that such a duty might not be readily borne.

What can we realistically ask of people? What can they realistically ask of themselves?[32] I want to put to one side those aspects of care which can be satisfying and those circumstances in which it works out well enough. They are by no means uncommon, and their possibility hardly out of the question. Moreover, I will say little here about the growing voluntary and informal groups and networks, as important as they are to the well-being of grown children and their parents.[33] I want to focus instead on those features of care which impose the sharpest moral demands on the caregiver, both to understand the dynamic of that situation and to see where government should be called upon for help. I have in mind particularly those circumstances which seem to pose a direct threat to the welfare and happiness of the person who gives the care, wherein the caregiver may become—by the sacrifice demanded and extracted—as much a victim of the illness or disability as the person who is cared for.

How might we best think of the moral situation of a child called upon to provide care for an aged, needy parent? Different diseases and conditions must of course modify any general answer, as must different social and familial circumstances. But a common thread is that of a person unfreely and unexpectedly trapped into providing a level of care well beyond that ordinarily demanded in family life or as a part of filial obligation. I use the term "unfreely" to indicate a lack of initial choice in providing the care. One is drafted by circumstances, and sometimes just as roughly and abruptly as sailors used to be impressed into the British navy. Most often it is a dutiful daughter who falls into this role.[34] It happens "unexpectedly" in the sense that the family relationship which imposes the moral demand was not originally envisioned as one that would make a radical demand upon the self. One feels oneself to be the victim of capricious and inexplicable bad luck. One is being asked to give of oneself in ways that would otherwise have been unimaginable, and unimaginably unacceptable had it been possible to spell them out in advance.

How do people react to that combination of circumstances? They are likely, most often, to feel anger that an unwanted fate has been visited upon them, an anger as often turned inward as toward the person who needs help. Why has this happened to *me*? Will I ever escape? Can anyone possibly understand what this costs me? The anger in turn often generates guilt, sometimes because the anger is aggressively turned toward the elderly parent—one who may be perfectly blameless but is, nonetheless, the cause of the problem; and sometimes because one feels one has failed oneself—failed, by reason of one's otherwise hidden anger and rebellion, to live up to a moral ideal, to what a child is supposed to owe a parent. That others do not notice the failure is beside the point. The conscience knows, and that is quite enough. One is at once, on the outside, a noble and giving person, gamely and lovingly facing up to adversity, and on the inside, one who rebels with hostility at the self-giving that is unfairly, even outrageously demanded.

Anger and guilt thus play upon each other, tearing at one's self-image and gnawing away at the bond between the child and the elderly parent. That such a combination of feelings should on oc-

casion produce fantasies about the death of the aged person is hardly
surprising. It is the perfect imaginative solution to the unwanted
moral burden of caring for another, at once decisively final in the
liberation it promises and utterly acceptable as a social solution.
"What a blessing," they say, "that he finally died." It is understood,
though unspoken, that the caregiver too has been relieved by the
death. No more ideal a resolution can offer itself to the conscience.
But until that relief occurs—and it may not occur for years—the
conscience is all the more burdened. It seems almost a form of
murder to have such thoughts. But how could one not have them?

Then there is the question of prognosis. How long will this go on?
Uncertainty of outcome is one of the great burdens of parental care.
Has the loving, or at least enduring, child (but now an adult) been
sentenced to what may seem like life imprisonment, or to a short
term only? Not knowing the answer to that question can place one
on an emotional seesaw of grand proportions, tempted one day to
see progress in the faintest signs of improvement and no less tempted
the next to see no evidence of improvement whatever. At stake here
is the possibility of hope. All things may be endurable if the demands are limited, finite in depth and time. But a future that offers
no exit at all, even if the burden on a daily basis is not utterly
overwhelming, can be an obvious source of sadness and depression.
No burden can be greater than trying to imagine how one can cope
with a future that promises no relief. That is the very meaning of
despair and why it is the greatest, the ultimate human misery. If
time is (so it is said) the cure for unrequited love, it can be a curse
for that requited love which binds us to someone for years as a
caregiver.[35] Is that fair, and can so much be asked of us?

It is *not* fair, but can, for all that, be asked of us. As suggested
above, the particular nature of the family bond is not nearly so
important as a special feature of the relationship, that of the neediness and vulnerability of the family member who requires care.
Someone other than the child could, of course, provide care. But an
important aspect of the vulnerability of ill or disabled elderly *family*
members is that they may want, and surely sometimes need, the
kind of intimate, familial care that only someone close to them, an
integral part of their life and history, can provide. Caretakers are not
utterly interchangeable. An elderly wife needs her husband to care

for her, not just anyone. He is the one who once chose to cast in his lot with her and took the trouble over the years to come to know her in a way that is not likely for another. So too will an elderly parent usually choose a child for help. There is no reason another should be so concerned about his or her welfare. However humiliating it was for him, my father wanted me to change his bedpan for him as he was dying; not a trained nurse, who could have done a much more graceful job.

Vulnerability most requires a response from someone who deeply cares, someone who will remain faithful—but faithful to us as a special and distinctive person, not as a mere object of moral duty or universal love. As Michael Ignatieff has wonderfully noted in *The Needs of Strangers*, our mere human needs as such—for clothes, or food, or warmth—say nothing about our individuality. "There is no identity," he writes, "that we can recognize in our universality. There is no such thing as love of the human race, only the love of this person for that, in this time and not in any other. . . . Woe betide any man who depends on the abstract humanity of another for his food and protection."[36] All of this is simply to say that at the heart of any significant moral obligation is the vulnerability and ultimate neediness of another and, in the context of family life and illness, a vulnerability that often can fully be responded to only by a family member.

Yet even if we grant that an elderly family member can desperately need the care of another, and *only* that other can respond to the need in a fully adequate way, does that automatically entail a right on the part of the sick person to such care, and a corresponding obligation of the child to provide it? There is surely some considerable social agreement that if the demands are not great or excessive, some obligations do exist: parents ought to care for their ill children, husbands for their ill wives, and children for their elderly ill parents. Minimal decency seems to require that. But the idea of unlimited self-sacrifice on the part of the caregiver, in a time of rapidly increasing life expectancy and chronic illness, encounters heavy, and perhaps mounting resistance. One line of objection is primarily practical: the placing of excessively heavy burdens on people is simply unwise. They may well collapse under the pressure, and perhaps in the process actually increase the problems of those for whom they are supposed to care. It could be foolish to advance family care as social policy if the net result would be a sharp increase in divorce among elderly couples, physical and mental abuse of elderly parents by their caretaker children, widespread neglect, and other evidence of demands too severe to be widely borne. That could be a valid objection, although one ought not accept it too easily before seeing whether ways could be found to mitigate the burden.

I am, however, more interested in noting another line of objections, those which focus on the morally reasonable demands of self-love and self-interest as a way of establishing the limits of obligation. Contemporary moral philosophy, for instance, shows considerable nervousness about extending the scope of moral obligation much beyond explicitly understood and accepted contractual agreements.[37] To count as moral at all, an action must stem from a free choice; autonomy is an underlying requirement. The idea of noncontractual moral obligations, those forced upon us without our willing it, becomes highly problematic. They fall into the realm of the heroic and supererogatory—commendable and virtuous and edifying, but not *required* in the name of morality. Only duty can lay strict requirements on us, and it is not clear, as noted above, just what our strict duty to our parents is. The purpose of drawing such a sharp line is not necessarily to aggrandize the self or lead it into the green pastures of unfettered self-interest. It stems instead in great part from the philosophical difficulty of establishing a rationally defensible moral basis for involuntary self-sacrifice. Prove to me in an irrefutable way, the philosopher might say, that I must sacrifice my happiness and my welfare to care for my parents. That would not be easy to do.

Feminism has over the years been particularly concerned to combat a culturally reinforced trait of women to all-too-readily embrace self-sacrifice and a selfless life. Since women are the heavily dominant majority of family caregivers, that critique has a special importance. From another point of departure, Protestant theology since World War II has tried to find a better fit between the central Christian virtue of love of others and the more modern insights into the value and necessity of love of self. In particular it has had to take a more critical stance toward the idea that love must, of its nature, be selfless, wholly other-directed.[38] How, many came to ask, can one love another with openness and integrity unless one loves oneself also in some significant way?

Even if we agree that a decent love of self is a necessary foundation for the love of others, that does not tell us where a line might be drawn. One feminist writer, Judith Tormey, distinguishes between occasional self-denial and self-sacrifice. The latter she defines as "a special form of self-denial. It requires that the self-denial be for someone else's benefit, and in addition that one give up those things to which one has a right."[39] Yet if we do have a right to some things, it is not egoism to refuse to give them up on behalf of another person. "To be an egoist is, essentially, to be selfish. One need not be self-sacrificing, however, to be unselfish. To be unselfish one need only give the interests of others their proper weight."[40] That strikes me as a perfectly sensible statement, but also, for our discussion, perfectly useless. What we do not know is the weight we ought to give the neediness and the vulnerability of those elderly who require (or at least desperately want) family care. If their condition is serious enough, their deficits crippling enough, could their needs not then always seem superior to those of the able-bodied person caring for them? Their moral claims would, so to speak, always trump ours.

That problem has been remarkably neglected in writings on the elderly. We must look elsewhere for helpful insights. Stephen Post, a theologian, has explored the closely analogous issue of limits of parental obligations to impaired newborns and children. The need there is as stark as that of the frail elderly parent. Post suggests some possible limitations to what he calls "radical forms of self-denial for the good of others": (1) the interests and needs of third parties—for instance, other children and family members; (2) the avoidance of "melancholy and introspective self-obsession"—that is, a situation wherein the "self-denial suits the purpose of the agent rather than the beloved"; (3) a limitation for the sake of the child herself (or himself), who could have a legitimate interest in not wanting to impose in an "undue" way or "to hold a total blank check on others to their possible detriment"; and (4) a rejection of that form of selflessness which depends upon the other for "one's own self-definition." "Proper self-love," he notes, "is not to be confused with selfishness, nor should it be denounced as such."[41] The upshot is that "if a mother refuses the option of sustained self-denial in radical form on the basis of her appeal to self-identity, such refusal should not be dismissed." Well, perhaps not, but just what is there about her identity, and presumably the needs that go with it, that give them a moral weight superior to the welfare of her child? We are not told, presumably because there is no good answer to a question of that kind. A similar question could well be raised in the case of a child who claimed his needs took precedence over those of the needy parent, and that the parental needs were unexpected and thus outside the circle of filial obligation. Why?

Why should those who need our care—who are vulnerable in a way that only *we* can properly respond to—be said to forfeit their claim simply because we did not expect them to have such great needs? In the case of creating a child, it is certainly a foreseeable possibility; and our procreative actions directly bring about that possibility. It is no less a possibility that one's parents may come to be frail and chronically ill, even if one does not expect that to happen. That our parent's condition is, unlike procreation, not of our doing does not mean our parent will need us any the less. That life often does not turn out the way we plan and expect is not a sufficient reason to disavow possible obligations. It is the welfare and the good of the other that are the point of the commitment, and it can never be fully known in advance what that will require. Love and commitment would seem to be thin and fragile notions if they require predictable outcomes to retain their validity.

It is, however, far easier to point out the problems in most attempts to set limits to obligation than it is to offer a satisfactory alternative. Why is it so hard to do so? The most obvious reason is that it is difficult to generalize about the capacity of people to take on heavy moral burdens. Some children do wonderfully in caring for elderly parents, but others do not. Not all people seem equally able to give to others or to have the emotional strength to do so, even with the best will in the world. Some elderly parents are pleasant and grateful for the help they receive; others are not. We cannot, therefore, readily establish any set of reasonable expectations of

caregivers when heroic, extraordinary caregiving is needed. By definition, extraordinary needs require extraordinary moral resources,
and not all, or even most, people have them.

Is there a way out? Heroic self-sacrifice may be possible only if
understood within the context of an entire way of life, one that
honors and supports us as we try to bear what would otherwise be
insupportable demands. If it is the vulnerability of others that is the
source of their claim on us, the fact that we and only we can provide
the care they need, a care that responds to them as unique individuals and not merely needy examples of *Homo sapiens*, then we need
to find both inner meaning and external support. That we are called
upon to respond to someone else's vulnerability means that we, in
turn, become vulnerable also. Something is going to be taken from
us as the ineluctable price of self-giving, perhaps something as central as our hopes and our identity. What can be offered in return?
Those who do the caretaking of the frail elderly must themselves be
cared for.[42] They cannot themselves be left in self-sacrificial isolation. Our burdens must be pooled and shared. I can conceive of
myself making a radical sacrifice for another if I live in a community,
and am part of a way of life, that understands the interrelationship
of our mutual needs and vulnerabilities and creates social institutions to respond to them. It is precisely because life so often fails our
expectations that we need each other—to soften the blow, to spread
the burden, to help us explain our sorrows to each other. It is
precisely because the moral demands to give of self can be so outrageous, so utterly devastating, that we need to know others are
prepared to do the same for us. As much as anything, I suspect, it
is the isolation of the moral claim to heroic action that is so intimidating in our kind of society. We cannot be sure that others will
sustain us, or that others would do likewise for us if our needs
became heavy.

What I am saying only underscores the widespread call for improved systems of social support for those who care for family members. They need the financial and psychological support of state and
federal agencies, and they need responsive, sensitive people to
counsel them, to give them help, and to give them respite. But that
may still not be enough. Even with adequate social support, we may
still be faced with tragedy, still be faced with moral claims that seem

to confront us with imperative duties which are, for all that, impossible demands. How are we to give meaning to those demands? There are two ways in which that can be possible. The first is the support of our friends and neighbors, those who understand what we are going through and provide encouragement, consolation, and affection. The second requires a community response. The care of another must be transformed from a stark and unpalatable moral demand borne in isolation to a satisfying moral vocation, one respected by the community and buttressed with a promise of return in kind when the caregiver eventually comes, as we all will, to need care.

A good society is one that finds ways to avoid requiring too much heroism; it will seek to match needs and strengths. Most critically, it will be one that cares not only for the public harms visited on minority and other weak groups but also for the private harms that nature and life visit upon individual people. It was a collective and popular political decision over many decades to support the biomedical research and improved health-care delivery that are heavily responsible for the increase in the longevity of the elderly. The solution to problems generated by that decision should be no less collective. What is the basis of our collective obligation?

| The Moral Foundations of Public Policy

WHEN ONE LOOKS FOR THE MORAL and social foundations of public policy toward the elderly in the United States, no single or sharply defined focal point emerges. Traces of the classical idea of piety toward the elderly seem always to have been present to some degree, but regard for the elderly, which brought them respect and care, was from the first in America apparently mixed together with pragmatic motives: if the elderly were not cared for properly, they would become a burden upon the state. By the late nineteenth century, the economic viability of the middle-class family was seen in part as dependent upon protecting itself against the burden of kinship demands.[43] Common sense, not affection, dictated those premises for policy. As the historian David H. Fisher has noted, earlier Americans did not invest the elderly with great awe: they "received respect without affection, honor without devotion, veneration without love. . . . As time passed, old age became more exalted rather than less so—more honored, and yet less loved."[44] Perhaps it could hardly have been otherwise in a nation of immigrants, many of whom sought in America freedom from social no less than political oppressions, among them the power of the old over the young in more traditional societies. Frontier life favored the young and able more than the old and wise, and much of the violence and lawlessness of frontier towns stemmed from an excess of restless young males, lacking in wisdom but not in energetic deviltry.

Those immigrants, nevertheless, did, on the whole, bring with them a key social premise, which for some stemmed from the English Poor Law of 1601 or the Bismarckian social security system in the Germany of the late nineteenth century: that the needs of the elderly could go beyond the capacities of families to respond. It would then be proper and necessary for government to take on the responsibility for their care. Yet there was always some nervousness about that idea in the American context. Would not government assistance hinder self-reliance, or do harm to the family and its duties? The move from local programs—adapted to community values and needs and tied closely to family contributions—to the national programs of Social Security in 1935 and Medicare in 1965 brought that ambivalence to the foreground. National programs for the elderly have always rested upon somewhat shaky moral and legal premises; the elderly have been granted neither a natural nor a constitutional right to assistance. Congress remains free to expand or rescind benefits as it sees fit.[45]

Nor have the social security programs rested on a clear sense of mutual responsibility between the generations. The right of the elderly to government aid has usually been understood as in part an earned right, one meant to preserve economic security as recompense for a lifetime of labor.[46] Attempts to discern some higher morality in that arrangement, or the intimation of a covenant between the generations, yield uncertain fruit. Instead, as two historians have unsentimentally noted in an analysis of the 1935 Social Security legislation, "The general tone of the social security debates . . . was that of providing for those made dependent through no fault of their own and, more generally, for eliminating destitution as a factor that in turn could lead to social unrest and to disturbances in the general economic system."[47]

The foundations of the later Medicare program were, by contrast, perhaps more firmly rooted in a perception of need and its moral claims upon us than was the case in the earlier social security debates. Modern medicine has the power to save and improve life, yet can place health care out of reach for those living in poverty or even with a decent middle-class income. Only government-funded care can provide a basis of security against both the anxiety and the fact of illness in old age. At the base of that argument is an appeal to the needs and vulnerabilities of the old. Illness and debility will gradually rob many in old age, sooner or later, of the power of self-care, and few will have the ability to pay the high costs of health care at times of critical illness. That the elderly fall into such a situation is not their own fault. The health needs they have are part of their human, biological condition. We should respond to those needs because the old have no others to whom they can turn, and because we can see in them a vulnerability we will all eventually share. Their needs are, if we will only recognize it, our needs; we will soon enough be there ourselves.

Occasional deference has also been accorded in the justification of old-age policy to what might be called solidarity arguments, the moral bonds and interdependencies of the generations. As one prominent advocacy group for the aged has pointed out, "Because of the interdependence of generations, all generations have a common stake in social policies and intergenerational transfers that meet needs across the life course."[48] A related idea is that of "veteranship." There the stress is placed upon the contributions and sacrifices made by the elderly. In the words of Douglas W. Nelson, "veteranship . . . sees the past history of older persons largely in terms of working, investing, building, parenting, nurturing, teaching, soldiering, enduring. Given this perception, old age becomes a kind of compensation, an earned status. . . . Old age . . . is the occasion for repayment by the larger community."[49]

Whether the strongest foundations of social policy for the aged are ultimately to be found in need, veteranship, or intergenerational reciprocity, it is clear they are bound together in practice with other motives as well. These motives include, among others: the self-interest of the young as they look toward their old age; the desire of the young to be spared the full weight of caring for their elderly parents; the aim of prudent government to avoid being saddled with an even worse economic burden if some early relief is not afforded the old; moral motives of respect and affection for the elderly; and a sense that a decent community should protect its weak, its frail, and its vulnerable from the ravages of old age. Any one of those motives might be sufficient to provide the impetus for government programs. Yet they are not all of a kind. When jumbled together, as they are in practice, such programs can generate profound uncertainties. The health that science can conceivably make available is unlimited in scope, as is the possibility of spending money in its pursuit. Are we really required as a long-term, open-ended commitment to say, as did Congress in 1965 in the Older Americans Act, that the old are entitled to "the best possible physical and mental health which science can make available and without regard to economic status"?[50] The morally problematic part of that commitment is to that "best possible" standard, one that has turned out to be without discernible boundaries.

That issue aside, it now seems well understood by the public (if not by all elected officials) that enforced legal obligations of children for financial support of their parents, for their medical or welfare needs, are mutually destructive. They rob the parents of their independence and trap the children into a depletion of their own family resources. Ben Wattenberg quotes someone who nicely catches an important point: "We [older folks] don't like to take money from our kids. We don't want to be a burden. They don't like giving us money either. We all get angry at each other if we do it that way. So we all sign a political contract to deal with what anthropologists would call the 'intergenerational transfer of wealth.' The young people *give* money to the government. I *get* money from the government. That way we can both get mad at the government and keep on loving each other."[51]

The great increase in life expectancy provides a solid reason, if one was ever needed, for arguing that all of us collectively, through the state rather than the children of the elderly, should supply the elderly basic economic and medical support. Both parents and children legitimately want an appropriate independence, but not the kind that sunders their relationship altogether or makes it utterly contingent upon active affection. A balance is sought between that independence which enables people to have a sense of controlling their own destinies, and those ties of obligation and affection which are for each an indispensable source of solace in the face of a world that has little reason to care for them. A minimal duty of any government should be to do nothing to hinder, and when possible what it can to protect, those ties which give families their power to nurture and sustain their members. To exploit the child–parent bond by coercively taxing families to provide economic or medical support for their elder members would be to threaten them with great harm; and it would be an action that presupposed a stricter form of moral obligation of children to parents than can rationally be defended.[52] At the same time, it promises to rupture those more delicate moral bonds, as powerful as they are conceptually elusive, which sustain parents and children in their lives together. Such bonds do not necessarily rule out noncoercive financial incentives for children to care for their aged parents. But if such incentives are to receive such support, then considerable caution will be needed to guard against any exploitation of elderly parents by avaricious children. There are, I ruefully note, as many ways of corrupting the parent–child relationship as ways to sustain it.

| Fragments of a Synthesis

I HAVE SUGGESTED that there have been, historically, a variety of moral reasons advanced about why the young should respect and care for the aged. These include most notably their needs and dependencies, their veteranship, and the interdependence of the generations. Yet the mixture of those motives with each other and with others of a more pragmatic and occasionally self-interested kind leaves some incoherency and a lack of focus at the basis of our morality toward the aged. That begins to show most noticeably when we try to find the right balance between government and family aid, and between self-sacrifice for the elderly and the legitimate claims of children to their own lives in the face of parental needs. It may well be that no stable balance can be found. Constantly changing social, medical, and economic circumstances will probably always require shifts and adjustments and the use of sensitive, practical reason. Nonetheless, I want to attempt a brief synthesis.

1• The Needs of the Elderly and Their Claims upon the Young. That the young continue strongly to recognize the needs of the elderly seems indisputable, even if (one might surmise) a partial reason for this is their recognition that they want a society which will one day take care of them also. The primary need of the elderly is to have their vulnerability, their dependence, recognized and responded to when it makes its appearance. That need constitutes a powerful moral claim in its own right, one comparable in its power to the claim of dependent children upon their parents; it seems inescapable and undeniable. The young, that is, have a duty toward the elderly simply because the needs of the old are undeniable and sometimes only the young can respond to them.

Yet need alone is probably not a fully adequate, or satisfying, basis for determining the obligations of the young toward the old. The young must also recognize their debt to the past, and particularly to those who helped build that past from which they now profit. The venerable idea of piety toward the elderly, however strange its sound to modern ears, is still pertinent. The related idea of veteranship has a similar pull, suggesting the validity of respect for the concrete contributions of the old in years past. The problem with need alone as the basis of claims is its cultural abstractness, its tendency to level everyone to the elderly's weaknesses and vulnerabilities. By contrast, the classical idea of piety toward the elderly, and the more contemporary one of veteranship, add to "need" the important element of respect for the specific contributions of the elderly to the nurture of the society which the young now enjoy.

That emphasis in turn underscores the interdependence of the generations, each of which has its own contributions to make and its own history to offer. No society can exist, much less flourish, without that interdependence.[53]

There is no pressing necessity to choose among need, veteranship, and reciprocity as a moral and social foundation for care of and respect for the elderly. Need provides the strongest basis when it is a matter of responding to an elderly individual, for it will focus only on the deficits and requirements of the person before us; merit will not be a consideration. Need, moreover, as a foundation of social policy has the advantage that it will be equally responsive to the needs of the old and the young. The old can have similar needs to those of younger age groups in their requirements for minimally adequate levels of food, clothing, and shelter, and to have those medical needs met which threaten suffering or a premature death. Veteranship and reciprocity, by contrast, would provide the basis for a response to the elderly that focused on them as members of a group, not as individuals. It would, in the case of veteranship, look to the merits of the old in general as those who rendered valuable services to society in the past. Reciprocity also looks to the aged more as a group than as aged individuals, but its emphasis lies in the value, over time, of establishing ongoing bonds of obligation and mutual duty between the generations. It is not too fanciful, perhaps, to say that need points to the present situation of the aged, veteranship to the past, and reciprocity to the future. That formulation would suggest that a social policy rooted in a blending of the three possible moral foundations would be stronger than one which settled on one of them alone; and they are also mutually reinforcing.

2• *The Needs of the Old and the Needs of the Self.* Even as we recognize the duty of society to help the young in their care of the old, we should sympathize with the inner struggle that the young can have in determining just how far their moral duties require them to go. No earlier society had to cope with so many old people living such long lives. Society may well recognize in a general way that there should be boundaries to the demands of altruism and self-sacrifice on behalf of the elderly. But that awareness does not deliver to caregivers a sense of where they personally should draw the line, where they can legitimately claim their own needs and future; and it is the highly dutiful who, most typically, will anguish the most over that problem. Let it be said that they need not totally sacrifice themselves; but let it be said also that they may seem to be presented, in reality, with no choice but to do so (though as a male I am embarrassed by the fact that few men seem to see the moral necessity that women do in those circumstances—that can hardly be a coincidence).

That is the horror and tragedy for many children of elderly parents. There simply may be no one else in the whole world who can give what the parent needs. All we can do in that case is work toward a community which acknowledges those tragedies and which respects, and tries to help, those who must live with them, for the most part hidden from our sight. Then it is that friendship can help, others to whom we may turn for support. Then it is that government as well as voluntary community groups themselves can show they are willing to alleviate, even if it cannot obviate, the situation.[54] Then it is that we show our society as one which knows that the duty of the young to the old is a demanding duty, one that admits of little compromise, either in reducing or evading the needs of the old, or in escaping the demands that the old legitimately make upon the young.

3• *Government and Families.* Historically, it was families and children who first took care of the frail elderly. A sense of reciprocity between the generations was long a premise of the care of the old by the young, especially those in the same family. The advent of government assistance was a way of recognizing the greater needs of the elderly (and their greater numbers and longevity) and the necessity of finding some relief for overburdened young people forced to care for their parents. With the advent of the Social Security system, and then Medicare, that recognition was all the more formalized and adapted to contemporary realities. The most important of those realities is that most of the elderly must, at some point, cease working and, save for the most affluent, will most likely require financial assistance. Moreover, they will at some point most likely become ill and require expensive medical assistance. They cannot live out their years in dignity without such assistance. The young, whose task it is to manage the society and care for those in need, must come to their aid through the apparatus of government. No other feasible, or dignified, solution is available. Care of the aged must remain a fundamental duty of government.

But government cannot meet all needs, and in particular cannot meet the need for personal care of, and affection toward, the elderly. Only the young, in person and intimately, can do that (although paid home attendants can sometimes achieve a comparable relationship). Families thus remain critical in the care of the elderly; they must supply what the impersonal ministrations of government could not conceivably supply. That is only to say that the young should help each other in carrying out their mutual duties toward the old. The obligation of children toward elderly parents must be a limited obligation, at least for most people. It is the responsibility of society to recognize those limits and come to the aid of those whose elderly parents press upon them demands that only heroism could meet. Some heroism may be needed; but a steady diet of it is intolerable. At the same time, there should be little disagreement that a society in which the young fail to recognize their own heavy obligations to the elderly—even if some are implemented by the apparatus of government—would be inhumane, even dangerous. That judgment should remain in the back of our minds when we consider the problem of allocation of resources to the elderly. For if, as I will propose, limitation on health care for the elderly is a defensible idea, its purpose should *not* be to spare the young the care of the old. Its purpose must be to see that each age group gets what it truly needs to live a life appropriate to it, and to see that each age group gives to the others that which it alone can give.

5 | Allocating Resources to the Elderly

THE POLITICAL DECISION TO SHIFT the primary burden of health care and social security for the elderly from their children and families to government was one of great and still-unfolding consequence. While it by no means relieved children and families of most traditional obligations toward their elderly parents and relatives, the intent was to shift their weight from the economic to the affectional sphere. As it has turned out, however, the domestic burdens within that sphere can be heavy and at times overwhelming, and exacerbated by greater longevity and changing family patterns. Outside help has been sought. Nor have all financial pressures on families by any means been relieved, especially when long-term institutional care of elderly relatives is required; a need for still greater financial relief for families has emerged. As the number and proportion of the elderly have grown, the economic pressure upon government continues to increase at a rapid pace.

What is the extent of the government's obligation? Or, to put the matter more precisely, what is the extent of our common obligation as a society—using the instruments of government—to provide health care for the elderly? If we must acknowledge that the families of the elderly cannot meet all their legitimate needs, that there are limits to familial obligation, does that mean that the duties of government are thus unlimited? The only prudent answer to that question is no. Government cannot be expected to bear, without restraint, the growing social and economic costs of health care for the elderly. It must draw lines, because technological advances almost guarantee escalating and unlimited costs which cannot be met, and because in any case it has a responsibility to other age groups and other social needs, not just to the welfare of the elderly.

My purpose in this chapter and the next is to develop a rationale for limiting health resources to the elderly, first at the level of public policy (Chapter 5) and then at the level of clinical practice and the bedside (Chapter 6). Our common social obligation to the elderly is only to help them live out a natural life span; that is, the government is obliged to provide deliberately life-extending health care only to the age which is necessary to achieve that goal. Despite its widespread, almost universal rejection, I believe an age-based standard for the termination of life-extending treatment would be legitimate. Although economic pressures have put the question of health care for the elderly before the public eye, and constitute a serious issue, it is also part of my purpose to argue that, no less importantly, the meaning and significance of life for the elderly themselves is best founded on a sense of limits to health care. Even if we had unlimited resources, we would still be wise to establish boundaries. Our affluence and refusal to accept limits have led and allowed us to evade some deeper truths about the living of a good life and the place of aging and death in that life.

My underlying intention is to affirm the inestimable value of individual human life, of the old as much as the young, and the value of old age as part of our individual and collective life. I must then meet a severe challenge: to propose a way of limiting resources to the elderly, and a spirit behind that way, which are compatible with that affirmation. What does that affirmation mean in practice, and not merely in rhetoric? It means that individual human life is respected for its own sake, not for its social or economic benefits, and that individuals may not be deprived of life to serve the welfare, alleged or real, of others—individuals are not to be used to achieve the ends of others. To affirm the value of the aged is to continue according them every civil benefit and right acknowledged for other age groups unless it can be shown that their good is better achieved by some variation; to respect their past contributions when young and their present contributions now that they are old; and never, under any circumstances, to use their age as the occasion to demean or devalue them. That is the test my approach to allocation must meet.

The greatest social benefit now enjoyed by the American elderly comes from a social security system that provides a minimal level of financial maintenance and heavily subsidized health care. What those who designed the health portion of the system—beginning with Medicare in 1965—did not reckon with was that its high and ever-escalating costs could in the long run threaten its viability. Federal expenditures for Medicare, for example, have been projected to rise from $74 billion in 1985 to $120 billion in 1989—a 60-percent increase in only four years. The threat that escalating figures of that kind portend—an eventual need to scale down benefits and to reconceive health care for the elderly—seems a cruel blow to the gains that have so recently been achieved. It is a basic assault upon the dream of a modernizing, aging society: that old age and good health are biologically compatible and financially affordable.

Initially, the economic issues of health care for the elderly seem to present an array of issues that are difficult but not unfamiliar. Among them are cost effectiveness in the delivery of care, the fair allocation of resources, effective and affordable methods of insurance, and the establishment of priorities for research. Is there, then, any reason to think that the economic problems of health care for the old are unique? Similarities can surely be noted in the case, say, of caring for severely handicapped newborns or for other groups of patients wherein the interventions are exotic, the costs high, and the ultimate results often problematic. Yet the difficulties of caring for the elderly display three unique features. The first is the increasingly endemic nature of their illnesses, which are less curable than they are controllable. The price of an extended life span for the elderly is an increase in chronic illness. The second feature follows from the first: the sheer number and proportion of the elderly as a pool of ill or impaired people. The third is the growing necessity to make painful moral choices in the care of the elderly dying as a class, particularly among those who end their days incompetent and grossly incapacitated, more dead than alive.

Health care for the elderly encompasses, then, some features shared with other age groups and some that are unique. How should we, therefore, think about the allocation of health resources to the elderly? I want to approach that question from the moral perspectives I have laid out in earlier chapters. The main points to be included within such an approach are that the allocation of resources to the elderly should be based upon (1) suitable goals for medicine, by which I mean achievement of a natural life span and, beyond that, only the relief of suffering; (2) an appropriate understanding of the meaning and ends of aging, particularly in terms of the search for personal meaning coupled with service to the young and coming generations; (3) a commitment by the young to assist the elderly to achieve their end in dignity and security, but in a way compatible with the other familial and social obligations of the young and without placing excessive or unreasonable demands upon them; and (4) the achievement of a death by the elderly that is humane. To these points I would add two additional ideals not previously developed: (5) a deployment of economic and other resources oriented to the good of society and its different age groups, not simply to the health and welfare of elderly individuals; and (6) the goal of minimizing as far as possible economic and social anxieties about growing old and being old. This last point requires making credible the belief that in one's old age one will be treated with dignity and respect, be assured of minimally adequate welfare and health care, and be supported by society in one's effort to find meaning and significance in aging and death.

| Facts, Projections, Significance

I HAVE BEEN WORKING with the assumption that there is a growing problem of allocating health care to the elderly. There is enormous resistance to that idea. Is it true? As with any other definition of what is or is not a "problem," everything will depend on how we interpret the available evidence. Carroll L. Estes, for one, has suggested that the whole debate about the future viability of Social Security is a manufactured "crisis," one designed to delegitimate the elderly as a deserving group. Reality, he argues, is being defined to make old age and an aging society a problem; thus can the elderly be "blamed for their predicament and for the economy" and domestic spending reduced as a consequence.[1] That is not a wholly farfetched idea and might be applied to Medicare as well as Social Security. Yet what are the available facts and projections about the health-care needs of the elderly? How reliable, in particular, are the projections for future needs? What is the significance of those projections, and in what sense do they indicate a problem?

The basic facts of the present situation can be briefly summarized. In 1980, the 11 percent of our population over age 65 consumed some 29 percent of the total American health-care expenditures of $219.4 billion. By 1984, the percentage had increased to 31 percent and total expenditures to $387 billion. Medicare expenditures reached $59 billion in 1984, while Medicaid and other government health expenditures on the elderly came to an additional $15 billion. Taken together, these government programs covered approximately 67 percent of the health outlay of the elderly (compared with 31 percent for those under 65).[2] Some 30.1 percent of the elderly classified their health as fair or poor in 1981, with some 45.7 percent of that number reporting some limitation of activity due to poor health.[3] In 1984, personal health-care expenditures for those 65 and older came to a total of $4,202 per capita (in comparison with $1,785 in 1977).

Projections for the future are less certain, but some typical figures are as follows. Between 1965 and 1980, there was an increase in the life expectancy of those who reached age 65 from 14.6 to 16.4 years, with a projected increase by the year 2000 to 19.1 years. Between 1980 and 2040, a 41-percent general population increase is expected, but a 160-percent increase in those 65 or over. An increase of 27 percent in hospital days is expected for the general population by 2000, but a 42-percent increase for those 65 and over and a 91.2 percent increase for those 75 and over. The number of those 85 or older will go from 2.2 million in 1980 to 3.4 million in 1990 and 5.1

million in 2000; and those 65 and older from 25.5 million in 1980 to 31.7 million in 1990 and 35.0 million in 2000.[4] Whereas in 1985 the elderly population of 11 percent consumed 29 percent of health-care expenditures, the expected 21-percent elderly population will consume 45 percent of such expenditures in 2040. The distinguished statistician Dorothy Rice, on summarizing the evidence, has written that "the number of very old people is increasing rapidly; the average period of diminished vigor will probably rise; chronic diseases will probably occupy a larger proportion of our life span, and the needs for medical care in later life are likely to increase substantially."[5] Karen Davis, formerly director of the federal Health Care Financing Administration (HCFA), has stated that "Future demographic and economic trends will strain the ability of public programs to maintain the current level of assistance, and will further magnify the gaps. Even with the uncertainties of technological change, biomedical research, and health-related behavior of the population in future years, it seems safe to predict that the gap between expanding health-care needs and limited economic resources will widen."[6]

Need we accept the judgments of Rice and Davis, or of others who believe (as I do) that the projections point to a grave problem? There are some who think the whole debate that is emerging over the costs of health care for the old, and particularly the possible strains it might create between the generations, is misplaced. There are also a few who think that one reform in particular, a control of useless and expensive care in the case of the dying elderly, would provide major economic relief. These reservations are serious and deserve reflection. I want to look at four general lines of criticism of the belief that there is a "problem" as well as to examine the view that the elimination of excessive spending on the elderly dying would be the single most efficacious way of reducing the health-care costs of the elderly.

1• The Heterogeneity of the Old and Long-Term Projections. Two objections to any supposed need for rationing are frequently joined. The first is that it is a mistake to allow future projections based on extrapolations from present data to dominate our thought, as if projections could give us an accurate picture of the future, or as if the future were immutable, not subject to policy manipulation. The second is that it is no less a mistake to think we can make illuminating projections about the aged as a group. They are too diverse to make that a meaningful exercise. It also contributes to a stereotyping of the old and a consequent failure to attend to the specific needs of specific individuals and subgroups among the aged.[7]

All projections into the future are, to be sure, uncertain, especially in the case of societies that change as rapidly as the United States. Yet as a general rule, there is no other way to plan for the future than to make extrapolations from present trends. That they may turn out to be wrong, or may be subject to great variation, is no good reason to evade the responsibility of making them in the first place. In the case of the aging, moreover, the palpable vastness of the demographic changes now taking place, their undeniably great implications for social and personal planning, and the harmful possible consequences of not having some kind of strategy (however tentative) for dealing with them would seem flagrantly irresponsible and irrational. While past projections about health-care needs and costs concerning the elderly have been wrong, they were almost always *underestimates* of mortality and morbidity trends and of health-care costs.[8] Two trends in particular were underestimated: that of life expectancy beyond the age of 65, and that of the number and proportion of those over 85. The health-care costs of the latter have become particularly pronounced. There is, more generally, little room to doubt that the number and proportion of the elderly are growing rapidly at present, that the number of young people in the demographic pipeline ensures a continuing growth of the elderly in the future, and that the old have greater health needs than the young. That is a trend which cannot be ignored; and there is no reason whatever to believe it will be reversed. Even if the inflationary costs of health-care delivery generally can be controlled, the combination of steady-state general costs combined with a growing pool of aged would guarantee a substantial increase in costs of care for the elderly. In the meantime, of course, health-care costs continue to outstrip the pace of inflation, so far impervious to cost-containment remedies.

The objection that the old are too heterogeneous a group to allow for any meaningful generalizations raises more serious problems. It incorporates both a technical issue (the validity of statistical or other generalizations) and a value-laden policy issue (the moral and social implications of categorizing people on the basis of their age and not merely their needs). Regarding the technical issue, while it is true that the aged are a remarkably heterogeneous group—and generalizations or predictions about any given elderly individual difficult to make—that does not mean group generalizations of some soundness cannot reliably be made. Many groups of people are heterogeneous, displaying a wide range of personal traits along a broad spectrum. But both because our language requires the use of general terms if we are to communicate at all, and because moral and policy considerations force some degree of generalization, there is no escaping the use of broad terms regardless of individual variation.

We know, for instance, that people over the age of 65 have greater health-care needs as a group than those under 65, that they are more in danger of death, that they are less suitable for physical-contact sports, that they tend to look different from those under the age of 10 (in ways that can be well characterized). That there are border-line disputes about just which age should be called "old" (whether 65, or 75, or 80) hardly proves that the word "old" is a meaningless category. It is simply a category encompassing great diversity and open to dispute. Many general and socially necessary terms (as an instance, "adolescence") have the same characteristics; that just means some care is required in using them, not that they should be dismissed altogether.

There would be little concern over these linguistic matters but for their political and moral implications. A concern about stereotyping typically underlies the wariness toward generalizations about the old: that they will be thought of as homogeneous, and in harmful ways. Some of that wariness has, of late, also been urged on advocacy groups for the aging. They have been accused, in the name of publicizing the problems of their constituents, of exacerbating a public image of the old as uniformly weak, frail, and poor. A newer stereotype of the elderly as affluent and pampered is no less rejected.[9] The worry about stereotyping is certainly legitimate. Yet many true generalizations about the elderly that are not offensive stereotypes can be made, particularly about their health status *as an age group* in comparison with other age groups. No general statement, however true in general, will be exactly true about any given individual. That does not invalidate their general truth. To say that the aged have greater health-care needs than other age groups is true. To say that death comes to all the old is also true.

Generalizations are also politically necessary. Since many of those most concerned about the stereotyping of the old are those who have worked hard on their behalf, their own cause would be threatened by a successful effort to eliminate all group generalizations. There are also related hazards in making too many distinctions about the aged and overstressing their heterogeneity. An excessively large number of subcategories of the aged, one way of coping with the diversity problem, could create bureaucratic and public confusion and could lead to competition among the aged themselves. The need for some coordinated political strategies on their behalf makes it therefore all the more important that the heterogeneity be of a recognizable general group: the elderly. Otherwise the sheer diversity of the needs and demands may confuse both government and the public.[10] The question is: For what purposes are we grouping and generalizing, and are they valid? An effort to focus exclusively on the needs of the elderly as individuals, rather than as members of a distinct group, is not a viable policy direction. It would threaten solid and helpful traditions that enhance respect for the elderly, would ignore perfectly valid generalizations about the elderly, and would force the pretense that age is a trivial or irrelevant human characteristic.

2• Is Rationing Necessary? In April of 1983, Roger Evans published a two-part article in the *Journal of the American Medical Association* with the title "Health Care Technology and the Inevitability of Resource Allocation and Rationing Decisions."[11] That article was by no means the first to stress the eventual need for rationing decisions, but by its emphasis on the "inevitability" of that development, it expressed a major (though hardly undisputed) trend in policy thought. The factors that produce the inevitability are an aging population, an increase in the prevalence of chronic disease, and the emergence of an array of expensive medical technologies to cope with those developments. "In short," he concluded, "the demand for health care will doubtless outstrip available resources."[12] In a much-discussed 1984 book, *The Painful Prescription: Rationing Hospital Care*, Henry J. Aaron and William B. Schwartz compared the British and American health-care systems to see what Americans might learn from the British about rationing, which they took to be inevitable also in the United States.[13] That the elderly are more subject to rationing in Great Britain than children or younger adults was one not-unexpected finding.

While it is difficult to gauge just what the present balance of opinion is among those in the health-care field on the need and justification for rationing of health care in general, two lines of objection have emerged. One of these is that even though the United States now spends close to 11 percent of its GNP on health care, there is nothing magical about that figure or any need to assume it should stay there or be lower. Why, it has been asked, could not the percentage go to 12 percent or 14 percent or 15 percent? That is theoretically possible, but it fails to take into account the important reality of political acceptability. That the United States already devotes a larger portion of its GNP to health care, 10.8 percent in 1986, than other developed countries with excellent health-care systems is itself a good reason for politicians and health planners to believe that more money would not in itself guarantee any greatly improved level of health care.[14] On what basis other than that might they persuade the public to tolerate a higher proportion of expenditures on health? While public-opinion polls often indicate a willingness on the part of the public to spend more money on health care, the apparent political perception is that there is little tolerance for greatly increased expenditures.

Another objection is that any talk of rationing is premature. The gerontologist Robert Binstock has said that future economic strains should not be blamed upon the elderly, but instead "lie in our unwillingness to confront and control the causes of runaway health care costs."[15] Others agree. Marcia Angell, Deputy Editor of *the New England Journal of Medicine*, has argued not only that more health care is not necessarily better care, but also that much present care is wasteful and unnecessary. This includes needless laboratory and diagnostic tests, "big-ticket" operations and procedures, and aggressive care of terminally ill patients.[16] Two other analysts contend that "evidence that rationing effective services in the United States may be unnecessary comes from three areas: the wide variation in per-person rates of use of all forms of medical care, the unproved effectiveness of many procedures used to diagnose and treat illness, and the unquestioned assumption among both medical practitioners and the public that doing more or at least doing something is preferable to doing nothing."[17] Another commentator, also stressing the inefficiencies and waste of the present system, has gone even further and contended that "invoking the language of rationing . . . has been at best, poorly thought through and, at worst, unethical."[18]

There can be little doubt that the present system is wasteful. The prospective-payment system based on diagnosis-related groups (DRGs) initiated in 1983 to control the costs of hospitalization under Medicare has shown that patients can be moved out of hospitals more quickly, and the proliferation of outpatient surgical and other medical procedures shows still other ways of reducing hospital costs. Research has demonstrated a striking variation from one community to another in the number of surgical procedures performed, a variation pointing to a lack of criteria for and control of necessary care.[19]

Nonetheless, despite some cost reductions here and there, there is so far no significant evidence that any striking savings of the kind envisioned by Binstock or Angell can, or at least will, in fact be made. Despite efforts dating back to the late 1970s to control or reduce health-care costs, they continue to rise in an uninterrupted fashion. Despite occasional claims that costs are beginning to come under control—*no one* has claimed that they are in fact already under control—the evidence is solid that health-care expenditures rose more rapidly after 1980 than earlier, and that relative to the overall consumer price index, more rapidly after 1980 than in the late 1970s. That trend continued with no abatement at all right through 1986.[20] Despite the politically inspired, and not implausible, belief that competition among providers would reduce costs, it seems instead to have raised them.

To look to theoretically possible efficiencies as a way out of our problems in caring for the aged thus seems to be wishful thinking with little historical or present basis. Even if *some* savings can be made, which surely is possible, new technologies are constantly being introduced that drive the costs higher, and technologies originally introduced to help the young are extended to care of the aged. Heart transplants, for instance, have now been extended to patients in their 60s, and a liver transplant was successfully carried out on a 76-year-old patient in 1986. As late as 1980, such patients would have been considered too old. Medicare was extended in 1987 to include heart and other organ transplants.[21] With an aging population, there will be an ever-larger pool of candidates to use those technologies—hardly a recipe for cost reduction. The evidence, on balance, suggests the need both to "cut the fat" (as the most common expression has it) and to ration as well. To depend on the former's doing a sufficient job in time would seem an act of unjustified faith; while to depend on the latter without strenuous efforts at the former would seem harsh and unfair. No one has been known to suggest that we could spend less money in the future on health care, either in real dollars or as a percentage of GNP; it has been suggested only that we might not have to see continued high growth rates. Moreover, while we might imagine a great change in the direction of stabilized or reduced costs, or simply muddling through with higher costs, that still leaves open the question I have been pressing: even if we can find the money, and avoid rationing, are large expenditures on health care for the elderly a wise way of allocating resources? That question is rarely if ever addressed in discussions of ways to avoid rationing or by those intent on denying its need.

3• *Guns or Canes?* An important variant on the objections to the need for rationing of health care is what has been called the "guns versus canes" argument.[22] It has a number of versions. If we can afford to spend more than $300 billion on national defense each year (much of it notoriously wasteful), another $25 billion on tobacco products, and $500,000 for a Super Bowl commercial, why should we entertain at all any serious discussion of cutting back or holding down expenditures on the sick and the elderly?[23] A heavy focus on the costs of care for the aged may simply serve to divert attention from other costs that are far less acceptable. Another version—in response to data supposedly showing that the elderly are benefiting more from government programs than the young—holds that even if this is true, it would be foolish for advocates of the aged to reduce their demands as a way of benefiting children. There is no guarantee whatsoever in our political system that any savings on the old would actually be transferred to children. Why risk a sacrifice of the needs of the aged in a circumstance of that kind?

These are potent arguments. The lack of any coordinated health, welfare, and social planning means that each group has powerful incentives to pursue its own interests, even if it is known that other valid interests exist. They each have little reason to believe their interests would otherwise be fully acknowledged or that any sacrifice on their part would be met by similar action on the part of other interest groups. We lack a system designed to be a just way of allocating scarce resources, either within the health-care system itself or between health and other social needs. There thus seems to be no good reason for any one group to forgo its demands and needs in favor of other groups, at least if the motive is to help the other groups.[24]

There are some problems with that approach. It serves all too readily to encourage some diversionary thinking of its own, turning attention away from a full and candid evaluation of the real needs of the elderly and the costs of meeting them. The fact that worse economic villains can be found, or more foolish expenditures in other realms discovered, provides no justification for avoiding that self-examination. More fundamentally, one of the prices of living in a democracy is that people are allowed to have other needs and interests than those of health and health-care delivery. A goodly number of Americans, patently enough, want to spend large amounts of money on national defense, and cosmetics, and wasteful advertising. One can complain about that, and label the present policies as stupid, narrow, and self-interested or self-indulgent. I am prepared to do so. One should also work politically to correct the situation and not be willing to settle for the status quo. I am ready to join that cause. But it is in the nature of our political system to tolerate such harms until peaceably and democratically changed.

Even within that democratic context, however, if one group pursues its needs with single-minded zeal and achieves excessive success, that increases the likelihood that other groups will not get what they need. In theory there is no zero-sum game in a country as affluent (at the moment) as ours, but the political reality includes a limit to the tolerance of taxpayers. They will not pay equally well or generously for everything. A practical consequence of the large amounts of funds now going to the elderly (together with the strong political support they enjoy) is to make it highly likely that new funds will not be appropriated for the young or for other social needs; it is the economic status quo (which includes high defense spending) that will have priority. We then end with a painful paradox. A reduction of spending on the elderly in no way guarantees that the money saved would be spent wisely or well. But an escalation of spending on the elderly almost ensures that money will not be adequately available for other needs, including those of children. The fate of Medicaid, ironically, perfectly illustrates this truism. Whereas it was originally designed to provide general health care for the poor, its originally incidental inclusion of long-term care of the elderly has meant that as the latter's costs have risen, funds for the other poor have proportionately declined (to only 40 percent), driven down by the costs of long-term care.

4• *The "Common Stake" in Care for the Old.* While the subject of allocation of resources among the generations will receive further discussion in my last chapter, it is pertinent to touch on it in this context. The argument has been made, in effect, that there is no real problem of allocation of resources to the elderly for two important reasons. The first is that because everyone either is already old or will become old, a social policy of expenditures on the elderly benefits all generations in the long run; that is our "common stake."[25] Second, health-care benefits for the aged have some immediate value for younger generations. They help relieve the young of burdens of care for the elderly they would otherwise have to bear. Research on those diseases which particularly affect the elderly has the side benefit of frequently producing health knowledge of pertinence to the young and their diseases. It also promises the young relief, when they are old, from diseases which they would otherwise be forced to anticipate. They are reassured about their own future to a greater extent.

That is a plausible viewpoint. Called, in one of its variants, the "life course perspective," it "clarifies the reciprocity of giving and receiving that exists between individuals and generations over time."[26] Yet it also obscures some important considerations. It is a view that could be taken to imply that any amount of health care for the present old would be beneficial to society because it would benefit everyone else as well. If this is an implication, it does not follow. We must first and independently decide, in the context of comparison with other social needs, just how high a priority health care for the aged should have in relation to other social goods. Would too high a priority, with no fixed limits, be a sensible way to allocate health-care benefits in comparison with such other benefits as education, housing, or economic development? In the absence of such a determination, moreover, we could inadvertently do harm by gradually increasing health-care allocations to the present generation of aged (and those who will join them over the next decade or so), thus overpoweringly burdening with indebtedness the younger generations, guaranteeing that they could not, when old, have comparable benefits. We might, that is, establish a precedent of care and a financial debt for that care which could not be managed in the future.

If the aged proportion of the population promised to remain stationary over the next few generations, and *if* there were no great chance of any increase in the average life expectancy of the old or in the burden of chronic illness among them, and *if* the introduction of further life-extending technologies were unlikely—then, in that case, a "life course perspective" could be put immediately to work. But it cannot now rationally be used without the prior exercise of freshly deciding what we want old age to be, which kind and proportion of resources we ought to devote to old age, and what the long-range implications of our choices for both old and young may be. Precisely because the future of aging, medically and socially, is so open-ended, so subject to some conscious ethical and policy decisions, it would be a mistake to simply leap into the middle of an indeterminate "life course perspective." We have to fashion that idea anew, taking into account as a necessary first step some basic judgment about how much and what kind of health care would be right for the elderly in the future. A "life course perspective" does not obviate the need to determine appropriate health care for the elderly, but logically requires it (together with a similar determination for other age groups) as a first step.

5• *Costs of the Dying Elderly*. The suggestion has been made by a distinguished medical economist that control of the costs of the elderly dying would be a major step toward eliminating the excessively heavy health-care costs of that age group. "At present," Victor Fuchs has written, "the United States spends about 1 percent of the gross national product on health care for elderly persons who are in their last year of life. . . . One of the biggest challenges facing policy makers for the rest of this century will be how to strike an appropriate balance between care of the [elderly] dying and health services for the rest of the population."[27] It is understandable that the gross figure—1 percent of the GNP—attracts attention. There are few physicians and increasingly few lay people who cannot find in their own experience of the elderly some cases of seemingly outrageous and futile expenditures to keep an elderly person alive. Bills running into the tens of thousands of dollars are common, and those in six figures hardly rare any longer. That kind of personal experience has solid empirical support. Studies of Medicare expenditures have shown that some 25 to 35 percent of Medicare expenditures in any given year go to the 5 to 6 percent of those enrollees who will die within that year, and that the high medical expenses of those who die are a major reason that health-care expenditures of the old rise with increasing age.[28] In addition to Medicare studies, a number of other analyses of the care of the critically ill indicate that the costs of caring for those who die are often much higher than for those who survive, and that the elderly are of course a high proportion of those who die.[29]

There is less here than meets the eye. Two issues need to be disentangled. The first is empirical. What exactly do the financial data show, and do they suggest that substantial savings would be possible if expensive care were withheld from the elderly dying? The second is ethical. Even if large amounts of money are spent on the elderly dying, is it an unreasonable and unjust amount?

The available data, while they support the charge of high expenditures, reveal a complex problem. The pertinent studies, for example, are all retrospective in nature; that is, they show only after the fact that someone died that large amounts of money were spent prior to the death. They do not tell us whether the initial prognosis was that of a terminal illness, whether care was taken not to waste money, and whether less expensive options for equally humane care were available. The point about prognosis is the most important. Can physicians ordinarily (save at the last moment) *know* that an elderly person is dying and that further sophisticated medical care will do the patient no significant good? Apparently not. As one of the more important studies concludes: "Among nonsurvivors, the highest charges were due to caring for patients who were perceived at the time of admission as having the greatest chance of recovery. Among survivors, the highest charges were incurred by those thought to have the least chance of recovery. Patients with unexpected outcomes . . . incurred the greatest costs . . . For the clinician, the problem may seem hopelessly complex. Simple cost-saving solutions, such as withholding resources from the hopelessly ill or earlier transfer of those requiring only anticipatory care, are difficult to apply to an individual patient because prognosis is always uncertain."[30]

A no less important finding is that the high expenses at the end of life are not largely the result of aggressive, intensive high-technology medical care. A Health Care Financing Administration (HCFA) study showed that only 3 percent of all Medicare reimbursements (some 24,000 decedents) went to those who incurred charges greater than $20,000 in the last year of life. Even the use of a lower threshold figure—of charges greater than $15,000—showed only 6 percent (56,000 decedents) incurring such costs.[31] Thus the economist Anne Scitovsky was justified in concluding that "the bulk of Medicare reimbursements for all elderly patients who die is accounted for by patients other than those who received intensive medical care in their last year of life."[32]

The combination of data of that kind and the clinical difficulty of an accurate prognosis that a patient is actually terminal means that optimism about the possibility of large-scale savings is misplaced. The constant innovation in critical-care medicine, most of it expensive, could well nullify other economies in any case. An additional important implication suggests itself: there is little basis to the moral conclusion that the money being spent on the elderly dying is unjust or unreasonable, even if quantitatively disproportionate to the spending on other age groups. That the aged are, as a group, going to be more expensive to care for than other medically needy groups is inevitable, inherent in the aging process. The expenditures could be judged unreasonable or unfair only if there were evidence that money was spent more inefficiently on the aged dying than on other patients—and no such evidence exists; or that, in the face of a known prognosis of certain or highly likely death, resources were nonetheless expended as if that were not known—and there is no basis to support that kind of general accusation. It then becomes rash to conclude that the spending is unjust. Since more money will proportionately and inescapably be spent on the old than on the young, and more of the old proportionately are likely to die despite such care, it is hard to see what is prima facie unreasonable and wasteful about that situation.

Does that mean there is *no* economic or moral problem? Not necessarily. I want only to conclude that the charge of wasted, useless expenditure on care of the dying elderly cannot be supported. There is, actually, an even more disturbing outcome of the studies to be discerned, well articulated by Anne Scitovsky: ". . . if further studies bear out the tentative conclusion that the high medical costs at the end of life are due not so much to intensive treatment of clearly terminal patients but to ordinary medical care of very sick patients, this raises much more complex and difficult issues than have been discussed in the literature to date. . . . A consensus has gradually developed about the ethics of forgoing treatment for such patients for whom care is, in some real way, futile. But no such consensus exists for patients who, although very sick, might still be helped by various diagnostic or therapeutic procedures and whose days might be prolonged. Thus, if we ask whether the costs of care for this group are excessive, we face new ethical problems of major proportions."[33] She bases this conclusion on evidence that the sickest elderly patients are actually treated less aggressively than younger elderly patients, and that the largest costs turn out to be those of providing long-term home and nursing care for the very frail and debilitated (and often demented) elderly, costs that can well exceed their acute-care hospital and physician costs.[34] Perhaps better solutions can routinely be found to the problem of those clearly identified as terminal (different hospital routines, expanded hospice options, for example). Even so, we will still be left with that other but much larger group of elderly, those who are patently, though slowly, declining but not yet imminently dying.

| Setting Limits

I HAVE CONSIDERED five responses pertinent to the contention that there is a need to ration health care for the elderly; while each of them has a certain plausibility, none is wholly convincing: It is possible and necessary to generalize about the elderly. It is possible that benefits to the aged will not automatically benefit other age groups. It is not premature to take the idea of rationing seriously. It is not a mistake to consider limitations on health care for the elderly even if there continue to be other social expenditures that we individually think wasteful. And it is more wishful thinking than anything else to believe that more efficient care of the elderly dying could save vast amounts of money. All those objections reflect a laudable desire to avoid any future policies that would require limiting benefits to the aging and that would use age as a standard for that limitation. They also betray a wish that economic realities would be happily coincidental with a commitment to the unrestricted good of the elderly. That may no longer be possible. A carefully drawn, widely discussed allocation policy is likely to be one safer in the long run for the elderly than the kind of ad hoc rationing (such as increased cost-sharing under Medicare) now present and increasing.

How might we devise a plan to limit health care for the aged that is fair, humane, and sensitive to the special requirements and dignity of the aged? As noted in Chapter 4, neither in moral theory nor in the various recent traditions of the welfare state is there any single and consistent basis for health care for the elderly. The ideas of veteranship, of earned merit, of need, of respect for age as such, and various pragmatic motives have all played a part in different societies and in our own as well. The earlier presumption of a basic obligation on the part of families to take care of their elderly, rooted in filial obligation, has gradually given way to the acceptance of a state obligation for basic welfare and medical needs. While the need and dependency of the elderly would appear to be the strongest basis of the obligation, it has never been clear just how medical "need" is to be understood or the extent of the claim that can be drawn from it. Minimal requirements for food, clothing, shelter, and income for the aged can be calculated with some degree of accuracy and, if inflation is taken into account, can remain reasonably stable and predictable. Medical "needs," by contrast, admit of no such stable calculation. Forecasts about life expectancy and about health needs have, as noted, consistently been mistaken underestimates in the past. Constant technological innovation and refinement means not only that new ways are always being found to extend life or improve therapy, but also that "need" itself becomes redefined in the process. New horizons for research are created, new desires for cures encouraged, and new hopes for relief of disability engendered. Together they induce and shape changing and, ordinarily, escalating perceptions of need. Medical need is not a fixed concept but a function of technological possibility and regnant social expectations.

If this is true of medical care in general, it seems all the more true of health care for the aged: it is a new medical frontier, and the possibilities for improvement are open, beckoning, and flexible. Medical need on that frontier in principle knows no boundaries; death and illness will always be waiting no matter how far we go. The young can already for the most part be given an adequate level of health care to ensure their likely survival to old age (even if there also remain struggles about what their needs are). For the aged, however, the forestalling of bodily deterioration and an eventually inevitable death provide the motivation for a constant, never-ending struggle. That struggle will turn on the meaning of medical need, an always malleable concept, and will move on from there to a struggle about the claims of the elderly relative to other age groups and other social needs. That these struggles are carried on in a society wary about the propriety of even trying to achieve a consensus on appropriate individual needs does not help matters.

For all of its difficulties, nonetheless, only some acceptable and reasonably stable notion of need is likely to provide a foundation for resource allocation. The use of merit, or wealth, or social worth as a standard for distributing lifesaving benefits through governmental mechanisms would seem both unfair at best and morally outrageous at worst. We must try, then, to establish a consensus on the health needs of different age groups, especially the elderly, and establish priorities to meet them. At the same time, those standards of need must have the capacity to resist the redefining, escalating power of technological change; otherwise they will lack all solidity. The nexus between need and technological possibility has to be broken, not only that some stability can be brought to a definition of adequate health care, but also that the dominance of technology as a determinant of values can be overcome.

Need will not be a manageable idea, however, unless we forthrightly recognize that it is only in part an empirical concept. It can make use of physical indicators, but it will also be a reflection of our values, what we think people require for an acceptable life. In the case of the aged, I have proposed that our ideal of old age should be achieving a life span that enables each of us to accomplish the ordinary scope of possibilities that life affords, recognizing that this may encompass a range of time rather than pointing to a precise age. On the basis of that ideal, the aged would need only those resources which would allow them a solid chance to live that long and, once they had passed that stage, to finish out their years free of pain and avoidable suffering. I will, therefore, define need in the old as primarily to achieve a natural life span and thereafter to have their suffering relieved.

The needs of the aged, as so defined, would therefore be based on a general and socially established ideal of old age and not exclusively, as at present, on individual desires—even the widespread desire to live a longer life. That standard would make possible an allocation of resources to the aged which rested upon criteria that were at once age-based (aiming to achieve a natural life span) and need-based (sensitive to the differing health needs of individuals in achieving that goal). A fair basis for limits to health care for the aged would be established, making a clear use of age as a standard, but also recognizing the heterogeneity of the needs of the old within those limits.

Norman Daniels has helpfully formulated a key principle for my purposes: the concept of a "normal opportunity range" for the allocation of resources to different individuals and age groups. The foundation of his idea is that "meeting health-care needs is of special importance because it promotes fair equality of opportunity. It helps guarantee individuals a fair chance to enjoy the normal opportunity range for their society." A "fair chance," however, is one that recognizes different needs and different opportunities for each stage of life; it is an "age-relative opportunity range."[35] Even though fairness in this conception is based upon age distinctions, it is not unfairly discriminatory: it aims to provide people with that level of medical care necessary to allow them to pursue the opportunities ordinarily available to those of their age. Everyone needs to walk, for example, but some require an artificial hip to do so. It also recognizes that different ages entail different needs and opportunities. A principle of limitation is also implicit: "Only where differences in talents and skills are the results of disease and disability, not merely normal variation, is some effort required to correct for the effects of the 'natural lottery.' "[36]

Yet there are two emendations to this approach that would help it better serve my purposes. For one thing, moral and normative possibilities of what *ought* to count as "normal opportunity range" are left unaddressed. For another, the concept should be extended to encompass what I will call a normal "life-span opportunity range"— what opportunities is it reasonable for people to hope for over their lifetimes?—and we will need to know what *ought* to count as "normal" within that range also. For those purposes we will have to resist the implications of the modernizing view of old age, which would deliberately make it an unending frontier, constantly to be pushed back, subject to no fixed standards of "normal" at all. Otherwise the combination of that ideology and technological progress could make Daniels' idea of a normal opportunity range for the elderly as an age group and my concept of a life-span opportunity range for individuals intractable and useless as a standard for fair allocation among the generations. The aged, always at the edge of death, would inevitably have medical needs—if defined as the avoidance of decline and death—greater than other age groups. No other claims could ever trump theirs.

Those considerations underscore the urgency of devising an ideal of old age that offers serious resistance to an unlimited claim on resources in the name of medical need, and yet also aims to help everyone achieve a minimally adequate standard. For that purpose we require an understanding of a "normal opportunity range" that is not determined by the state-of-the-art of medicine and consequently by fluctuating values of what counts as a need. "Need" will have no fixed reference point at all apart from a technology-free (or nearly so) definition. Where Daniels uses the term "normal" in a statistical sense, it should instead be given a normative meaning; that is, what counts as morally and socially adequate and generally acceptable. That is the aim of my standard of a natural life span, one that I believe is morally defensible for policy purposes. Such a life can be achieved within a certain, roughly specifiable, number of years and can be relatively impervious to technological advances. The minimal purpose is to try to bring everyone up to this standard, leaving any decision to extend life beyond that point as a separate social choice (though one I think we should reject, available resources or not). Daniels recognizes that his strategy has the implication that it "would dictate giving greater emphasis to enhancing individual chances of reaching a normal lifespan than to extending the normal lifespan."[37] But I think that that implication, to me highly desirable, really follows only if taken in conjunction with some theory of what *ought* to count as a "normal opportunity range" and not simply what happens to so count at any given historical and technological moment. The notion of a natural life span fills that gap.

With those general points as background, I offer these principles:

1• Government has a duty, based on our collective social obligations, to help people live out a natural life span, but not actively to help extend life medically beyond that point. By life-extending treatment, I will mean any medical intervention, technology, procedure, or medication whose ordinary effect is to forestall the moment of death, whether or not the treatment affects the underlying life-threatening disease or biological process.[38]

2• Government is obliged to develop, employ, and pay for only that kind and degree of life-extending technology necessary for medicine to achieve and serve the end of a natural life span; the question is not whether a technology is available that can save a life, but whether there is an obligation to use the technology.

3• Beyond the point of a natural life span, government should provide only the means necessary for the relief of suffering, not life-extending technology.

These principles both establish an upper age limit on life-extending care and yet recognize that great diversity can mark the needs of individuals to attain that limit or, beyond it, to attain relief of suffering.

| Age or Need?

THE USE OF AGE AS A PRINCIPLE for the allocation of resources can be perfectly valid.[39] I believe it is a necessary and legitimate basis for providing health care to the elderly. It is a necessary basis because there is not likely to be any better or less arbitrary criterion for the limiting of resources in the face of the open-ended possibilities of medical advancement in therapy for the aged.[40] Medical "need" can no longer work as an allocation principle; it is too elastic a concept. Age is a legitimate basis because it is a meaningful and universal category. It can be understood at the level of common sense, can be made relatively clear for policy purposes, and can ultimately be of value to the aged themselves if combined with an ideal of old age that focuses on its quality rather than its indefinite extension.

This may be a most distasteful proposal for many of those trying to combat ageist stereotypes and to protect the deepest interests of the elderly. The main currents of gerontology (with the tacit support of medical tradition) have moved in the opposite direction, toward stressing individual needs and the heterogeneity of the elderly. That emphasis has already led to a serious exploration of the possibility of shifting some old-age entitlement programs from an age to a need basis, and it has also been suggested that a national health-insurance program which provided care for everyone on the basis of individual need rather than age (as with the present Medicare program) would better serve the aged in the long run.[41] Thus while age classifications have some recognizably powerful political assets, a consensus seems to be emerging—clearly contrary to what I propose—that need is a preferable direction for the future. "Perhaps," as the Neugartens have written, "the most constructive ways of adapting to an aging society will emerge by focusing, not on age at all, but on more relevant dimensions of human needs, human competencies, and human diversity."[42] While that is an understandable impulse, I think it cannot for long remain possible or desirable in the case of allocating health care to the aged.

The common objections against age as a basis for allocating resources are varied. If joined, as it often is, with the prevalent use of cost–benefit analysis, an age standard is said to guarantee that the elderly will be slighted; their care cannot be readily justified in terms of their economic productivity.[43] The same can be said more generally of efforts to measure the social utility of health care for the old in comparison with other social needs; the elderly will ordinarily lose in comparisons of that kind. By fastening on a general biological trait, age as a standard threatens a respect for the value and inherent diversity of individual lives. There is the hazard of the bureaucratization of the aged, indifferent to their differences.[44] Since age, like sex and race, is a category for which individuals are not responsible, it is unfair to use it as a measure of what they deserve in the way of benefits.[45] The use of an age standard for limiting care could have the negative symbolic significance of social abandonment.[46] Finally, its use will run counter to established principles of medical tradition and ethics, which focus on individual need, and will instead, in an "Age of Bureaucratic Parsimony. . . . be based upon institutional and societal efficiency, or expediency, and upon cost concerns—all emerging rapidly as major elements in decision making."[47]

These are weighty objections, and the hazards perfectly plausible. But all of them fail, or are sharply neutralized in their power, if the grounds for the use of age as a criterion for allocation are respect for the fundamental need of the elderly only to live out an adequate life span, and a recognition that medical need as a standard is utterly unworkable in any case in the face of technological advances. My principle of age-based rationing is not founded on the demeaning idea of measuring "productivity" in the elderly. The use of age as a standard treats everyone alike, aiming that each will achieve a natural life span, productive or not. Far from tolerating social abandonment, it will aim at improving care for the elderly, though not life-extending care. A standard of allocation rooted not in dehumanizing calculations of the economic value or productivity of the elderly, but in a recognition that beyond a certain point they will already have had their fair share of resources does not degrade the elderly or lessen the value of their life. It is only a way of recognizing that the generations pass and that death must come to us all. Nor does it demean the aged as individuals, or signal indifference to the variations among them, to note that they share the trait of being old. It is only if society more generally devalues the aged for being aged—by failing, most notably, to provide the possibility of inherent meaning and significance in old age (as is the case with the modernizing project)—that their individual lives are treated as less valuable. There is nothing unfair about using age as a category if the purpose of doing so is to achieve equity between the generations, to give the aged their due in living out a life-span opportunity range, and to emphasize that the distinctive place and merits of old age are not nullified by aging and death.

That a society could be mature enough to limit care for the aged with no diminution of respect, or could recognize the claims of other age groups without an implication that the elderly are less valuable than they are, seems rarely to be considered. By contrast, the motives I have been advancing reject not the elderly, but a notion of the good of the elderly based on pretending that death and old age can be overcome or ignored, that life has value only if it continues indefinitely, and that there is nothing to be said for the inherent value and contributions of the elderly as elderly. A society that adopts a wholly modernizing approach to old age must necessarily find the possibility of any limitation on care for the elderly a threat. It has robbed old age of all redeeming significance, and only constant efforts to overcome it are acceptable. To pick on the aged for "bureaucratic parsimony," to use Mark Siegler's term, would surely be wrong if done because they were perceived as weak and defenseless, a nice target-of-opportunity for cost containment. That is a very different matter from a societal decision that the overall welfare of the generations, the proper function of medicine, and a fitting understanding of old age and death as part of the life cycle justify limitation on some forms of medical care for the elderly.

| Setting Priorities

THERE IS NO TASK IN THE FASHIONING of health policy more intimidating than establishing priorities; yet that is close to the essence of even having a policy. A policy might most concisely be defined as a set of priorities for action and the allocation of resources oriented toward achieving a goal. In this case, we are looking for a policy of allocating resources to the elderly consistent with acceptable and appropriate goals for their health and welfare. I want to present the outline of an allocation policy and priority system. It will be based on age as a legitimate principle of allocation, and will focus—in setting health-care goals for the elderly—on the averting of a premature death and the relief of suffering. This will be an "outline" only, not merely because my purpose here is more to think through the broad implications of a new and different vision of health care for the aged than to present a blueprint, but also because time and experience will be needed to determine what it would mean in practice. A full policy plan would include detailed directions, for example, for determining priorities within basic biological research, within health-care delivery, and between research and delivery. That I will not try to provide. I can only sketch a possible trajectory—or, to switch metaphors, a kind of likely general story. But if that at least can be done in a coherent fashion, avoiding the most flagrant contradictions, it might represent some useful movement. I will, however, take up some implications of this scheme in my next chapter.

There are four elements in my outline, three of which I shall examine in the remainder of this chapter. The first is the need for an antidote to the major cause of a mistaken moral emphasis in the care of the elderly and a likely source of growing high costs of their care in the years ahead. That cause is constant innovation in high-technology medicine relentlessly applied to life-extending care of the elderly; it is a blessing that too often turns into a curse. Unless an antidote is effective, and can be found, no alternative to the present arrangement is likely to take hold. The second element is a need to focus on those subgroups of the elderly—particularly women, the poor, and minorities—who have as yet not been well served, for whom a strong claim can be entered for more help from the young and society more generally. The third is a set of high-priority health and welfare needs—nursing and long-term care, prevention—which would have to be met in pursuit of the goals I have proposed. The fourth element, to be taken up in the next chapter, is the withholding or withdrawal of life-extending care from some groups of elderly patients.

1• High-Technology Medicine: Finding an Antidote. The great advances in health care in recent years have come from developments in high-technology medicine. Once the infectious diseases had been controlled or eliminated, further improvements in health have heavily depended upon technology (although changes in lifestyle, particularly in the case of heart disease, have made a contribution also). If any strong reins are to be put on the costs of health care for the elderly, high-technology medicine is one important place to begin. Most of the technological advances of recent decades have come to benefit the old comparatively more than the young (as an instance, dialysis) and the older segment of the old more than any other (as an instance, critical-care units).[48] Those same advances have also been heavily responsible for the increase in life expectancy that developed after the 1960s and continues to the present—and for the steady increase in chronic disease that has accompanied that increase. Technology has also had an important role in the rise in health-care costs. In analyzing the 8.9-percent increase in the cost of health care in 1985, the Department of Health and Human Services traced one-fourth of it to an "increased intensity of care," a combination of greater use of technology and a higher proportion of aged patients. The other sources of the increase were basic inflation in the economy and additional inflation in the cost of medical items above the national inflation rate.[49] Thus even if medical and other forms of inflation had been controlled, intensified use of technology would still have increased costs.

Where there is now a powerful bias in favor of innovative medical technology, and a correspondingly insatiable appetite for more of it, that will have to be replaced by a bias in the other direction where the aged are concerned. The alternative bias should be this: that no new technologies should be developed or applied to the old that are likely to produce only chronic illness and a short life, to increase the present burden of chronic illness, or to extend the lives of the elderly but offer no significant improvement in their quality of life. Put somewhat differently, no technology should be developed or applied to the elderly that does not promise great and inexpensive improvement in the quality of their lives, no matter how promising for life extension. Incremental gains, achieved at high cost, should be considered unacceptable. Forthright government declarations that Medicare reimbursement will not be available for technologies that do not achieve a high, very high, standard of efficacy would discourage development of marginally beneficial items.

While it would now be cruel to terminate federal kidney-dialysis support for the elderly, dialysis represents precisely the kind of technology that should not be sought or developed in the future. It does not greatly increase the life expectancy of its users (an average of only five years), and for most, that gain is at the price of a doubtful or poor quality of life and an inability to achieve earlier levels of functioning.[50] That it was originally developed with younger patients (aged 15 to 50) in mind, but soon saw an age creep of great proportions (with some 30 percent—25,000—of those on dialysis now over 65), is another part of the story to be remembered for the future.[51] The appeal to the Congress that in 1972 underwrote the costs of dialysis was that it would save lives and at a relatively modest cost (the estimate was for a maximum expenditure of $400 million). It has surely saved lives, but not for long, and the more than 80,000 users now cost well over $2 billion a year.[52] More generally, as a result of third-party reimbursement systems (up through 1983 at least, prior to the Medicare Prospective Payment System enacted by Congress in that year) there was, in the words of two analysts, "a near-maximum growth rate in the demand for new technologies to treat the elderly."[53]

The attraction of new and improved technologies remains as powerful now as it was in 1972, and their use gradually spreads from the younger to the older patient. That phenomenon is now visible in the cases of mechanical ventilation, artificial resuscitation, antibiotics, and artificial nutrition and hydration, four technologies singled out by the Congressional Office of Technology Assessment (OTA) in its important 1987 study of life-extending technologies and the elderly. While each of them is obviously of potential benefit for any age group, the greater likelihood of a life-threatening illness among the elderly means that they will be the primary candidates for their use. A reasonable estimate is that between 1980 and the year 2000, there will be an increase in the number of elderly of 9.5 million. That is a powerful incentive to continue improving those technologies, improvements that will almost certainly—on the basis of the historical pattern—extend their application to ever-sicker categories of patients at ever-increasing costs.

Consider some of the technological developments in this context. Antibiotics that can, at relatively low cost, be taken orally or given by injection are at present joined by those which can be given intravenously, a more expensive procedure. Eventually they will also be joined by those which can be infused by an implantable pump, a far more expensive procedure still. The provision of food and water can now go from the spoon and fork to the nasogastric tube, and then to the relatively new and very costly total parenteral nutrition (TPN), the last at a cost of $50,000 to $100,000 a year. Mechanical ventilation, a mainstay in the care of many elderly dying suffering from pulmonary insufficiency, is no less an area of advancing technology, ever able to sustain more people by ever-more-sophisticated means—high-frequency ventilation (HFV), extracorporeal-membrane oxygenation (ECMO), and—still in the theoretical stage—peritoneal oxygenation and carbon dioxide removal, and an implantable artificial lung. Since removal from a respirator is among the most common life-sustaining-treatment decisions, an increase in the efficacy of this technology alone is likely to intensify the moral dilemmas in the care of the elderly dying; and it is hardly likely to reduce the costs of caring for such patients.

Much of the use of these technologies would be devoted not just to the most desperately ill, at great cost and the frequent perpetuation of chronic disability, but also to any patient who could benefit from them. That is the common pattern with new technologies. An obvious dilemma here is that most technologies will benefit the young as well and are developed with them often primarily in mind. If technological development is discouraged, will that not damage the health interests of the young, even their chances to avoid a premature death? That is a hazard, but its effects could be lessened by a technology assessment that examined whether, if it were developed for the young, its primary or disproportionate use might be among the elderly, and whether alternative means could be found to meet the needs of the young. I leave these as difficult problems for the trajectory I am proposing.

However important though admittedly hard it would be to inhibit the development of marginally beneficial technologies, the larger problem lies not so much in what have been called the "big ticket" items as in the high costs of much more routine diagnostic and therapeutic procedures. "Ordinary" medical care, which accounts for most of the high costs of the elderly, is in great part driven by the routine use of what are by now routine technologies. That some 33 to 50 percent of the costs of medical care can be traced to technology suggests that a sharp focus on them in the case of the elderly is in order. Unless they can promise a high efficacy also, their routine employment should be discouraged. A telling commentary on present practice is the statement that "High quality acute care is necessary for the successful health of elderly [oldest-old] patients. Indeed, 44 percent of all present health care expenditures for the elderly arise from acute-care settings."[54] The value of this acute care, the authors emphasize, is to save on long-term-care expenditures, although they do not present any evidence that this result is usually achieved. If it is true that the road to hell is paved with good intentions, it is no less true that the road to higher long-term costs is paved with claims of the eventual savings to be achieved by the use of expensive technologies. A policy of systematic skepticism toward technology-driven expenses in the care of the elderly would serve a useful dampening effect.[55]

2• Providing Equitable Security. The greatest fear about old age seems to be not death but frailty, the loss of independence and self-direction, declining mental capacities, and impoverishment. The failure of present entitlement programs to cope with the fear of impoverishment as a result of old age and attendant ill health remains as a major flaw in the system.[56] While the elderly as an age group are now relatively well off, with only some 12 to 14 percent below the poverty line, a figure of that kind needs to be looked at closely. Those who live alone, the very old, and minority groups are much more likely to be in or only slightly above the poverty category than other aged people. In 1984, more than 1 in 3 black women 65 and over lived in poverty, and more than 1 in 5 Hispanic women. Women as a group constituted 71 percent, about 2.3 million, of the elderly poor; and women at all ages are twice as likely as men to be poor.[57] That is an intolerable situation.

A point not often sufficiently stressed is the insecurity that the present system breeds, even for those who are at the start better off. Though only a minority of the elderly are now in the poverty or near-poverty group, no younger person can be sure he or she will not be in that group, and no older person, even if well off at the moment, can be assured that some medical catastrophe will not put him or her into the group as well. Stories of the economic devastation wrought by catastrophic illnesses—or simply chronic illnesses that last for many expensive years—can be found in almost any family now. In general, also, the elderly are under pressure to reduce their use of hospital care. The Medicare deductible of about $500 is now twice what it was in the early 1980s, and general out-of-pocket medical expenses now take a larger portion of the income of the elderly than they did before Medicare went into effect in the mid-1960s.[58] Of the average $4,202 per capita consumption of health care by the aged in 1984, some 75 percent was paid by third parties (Medicare, Medicaid, or private plans), with the remaining 25 percent being paid directly. That latter proportion seems bound to grow. The Medicaid requirement of impoverishment—and thus a forced spending down of income and divestiture of resources—as a condition for qualifying for nursing-home or long-term care is a nasty threat to a lifetime of work and savings and a perfect symbol of government-imposed dependence.

The elderly (both poor and middle-class) can have no decent sense of security unless there is a full reform of the system of health care.[59] It may well be that reforms of the sweeping kind implied in these widely voiced criticisms could more than consume in the short run any savings generated by inhibitions of the kind I am proposing in the development and use of medical technology. But they would address a problem that technological development does nothing to meet. They would also reassure the old that there will be a floor of security under their old age and that ill health will not ruin them financially, destroy their freedom, or leave them dependent upon their children (to the detriment of both). It is, in any event, almost certain that unless the costs of technology are controlled, this reform has little chance of succeeding. Full or improved coverage for the elderly poor has historically competed badly against escalating reimbursements for high-technology care to existing beneficiaries.

Many years will be required to bring about the kind of shift in values needed to change attitudes and practices pertinent to the provision of life-extending technologies to the elderly. That is the long-term solution. In the meantime, while we are working toward that goal, an intensified effort to provide better basic health-care coverage for the elderly will most effectively demonstrate that there is no lessening of commitment to their well-being. It is that move—and no other—which will neutralize the kind of threat posed by a restriction of life-extending care. I cannot responsibly propose to limit that kind of care without simultaneously proposing to improve other forms of care. I will be the first to object to any effort to deny life-extending care before the other reforms are well under way and assured of success. A denial of the one without the flourishing of the other would indeed be a grave threat to the elderly.

3• Priorities for Care. A societal decision deliberately to limit life-extending high-technology care for those who have lived out a natural life span is not meant to be a recipe for, or symbol of, abandonment. It is meant to be an affirmation of the diverse needs of different age groups and an acceptance of the inevitable place of death at the end of life. It can be a tolerable basis for social policy only if that policy strikingly seeks to provide the elderly with an honorable and bearable life in their remaining years. This will entail first working to avert a premature death, and then seeking to minimize pain and suffering.

Any attempt to specify a "premature death" must have a certain arbitrary quality. I define it as a death prior to the living out of a natural life span, something that would ordinarily occur in the early 70s but could extend through the late 70s to early 80s. It is the latter range I will use as the basis for my discussion here. This is actually a more liberal standard than that used by the federal Centers for Disease Control (CDC), which uses the concept of "years-of-life-lost" prior to age 65 in determining premature death. That concept came into use during the 1970s and was incorporated into the CDC's *Morbidity and Mortality Weekly Report* in 1982. A focus on conventional death rates, by simply counting deaths in the population, emphasizes deaths occurring in older age groups. The "years-of-life-lost" calculation, by contrast, highlights the potentially preventable mortality occurring earlier in life and permits a more precise focus for health-care goals. A variant of that method has shown, for example, that accidents are the leading cause of premature death, while cancer and heart disease (affecting older people) fall into second and third places. Heart disease, which remains the leading cause among all deaths, thus falls by this calculation to a lower place because it is not as significant a cause of premature death. Using 1979 as the base year for its calculations, one important study determined that the rank order of causes of years lost is: accidents, cancer, heart disease, perinatal abnormalities, homicide, suicide, congenital abnormalities, cerebrovascular disease, cirrhosis and chronic liver disease, and pneumonia and influenza.[60] Whether this or some similar method of reckoning is used, the first goal in care for the aged will be to go after the causes of premature death.

Beyond avoiding a premature death, what do the elderly need from medicine to complete their lives in an acceptable way? They need to be as independent as possible, freed from excess worry about the financial or familial burdens of ill health, and physically and emotionally positioned to seek whatever meaning and significance can be found in old age. Medicine can only try to maintain the health which facilitates that latter quest, not guarantee its success. That facilitation is enhanced by physical mobility, mental alertness, and emotional stability. Chronic illness, pain, and suffering are all major impediments and of course appropriate targets for medical research and improved health-care delivery.

Major research priorities should be those chronic illnesses which so burden the later years and which have accompanied the increase in longevity. They encompass, in addition to a number of physical problems (particularly multiple organic diseases), a variety of major mental disorders, including schizophrenia, affective disorders, various senile brain diseases, arteriosclerosis, and epilepsy. The OTA study of aging and technology centered on five chronic conditions endemic among the elderly, of which only the first receives any great public attention (or, for that matter, sympathy): dementia, which characterizes Alzheimer's disease—a source first of humiliation, then of a loss of basic human potentials, then death; urinary incontinence—also a humiliating condition and a malodorous symbol of the loss of physical control; hearing impairment—embarrassing, isolating, and frustrating; osteoporosis (thinning of the bones)—because of the greatly enhanced incidence of fractures, a source of constant fear and danger for the old-old in particular; osteoarthritis—painful, sometimes disabling, and pervasive (affecting 16–20 million elderly).

As with the correction of inequities in health care for the elderly, there is no guarantee that the necessary research and future amelioration of such conditions would be inexpensive. Even low-technology approaches to noncurable chronic problems can be enormously expensive if used by enough people; and some of the therapeutic solutions to some of the conditions are clearly of the high-technology variety (e.g., hip and joint replacement at an average cost of $50,000 to victims of osteoarthritis). The most troubling problems in that respect may well be posed by advances in rehabilitation. Even now, rehabilitation for stroke is labor-intensive, difficult, and often of uncertain outcome, and the moral dilemma of choosing those patients most likely to benefit often wrenching. While rehabilitation has in the past been thought of as a low-technology, a caring rather than curing, field, it is also moving in a technological direction and, simultaneously, working to rid itself of the reputation of indifference to and pessimisim about rehabilitation for the elderly.[61] The ongoing development of sophisticated prosthetic devices and computer-assisted methods of helping the partially paralyzed, paraplegic and quadriplegic do not promise to lower costs, and neither does their likely extension to use among the elderly. If such developments as these are even to be possible, it is hard to envision how they can financially coexist with continuing investment in life-extending treatments.

The prevention of illness has long been promoted as the best way in the long run to improve the health of the elderly (along with the health of everyone else) and to reduce health-care costs. Its primary virtue from any perspective is that it can help avoid a premature death and enhance physical well-being through an ordinary life span; illness and death would be pushed beyond the normal lifetime-opportunity-range boundary. That it will actually reduce costs is not, however, necessarily true as a flat generalization. Whether the sum total of the direct costs (to mount and implement a program of prevention) and the indirect expenses (time and other social resources) will equal the savings will vary from one disease category to another.[62] In some cases, moreover, it will be no more expensive to cure a disease than to prevent it—for example, the choice between bypass surgery and a preventive regimen for the hypertension that would have led to it.[63] "This means," Louise Russell has written, "that choosing investments in health is more difficult than some of the claims for prevention would suggest. Sometimes prevention buys more health for the money; sometimes cure does. . . . the issue most often is what mix of prevention and therapy is best. It is a rare preventive measure that, like smallpox vaccine, eradicates the condition altogether."[64] Yet even if economic savings are uncertain in each case, prevention programs can have many health benefits, helping to avoid some conditions altogether (cancer most notably through such changes in behavior as the cessation of smoking) and ameliorating the impact of others (as in a reduction of obesity among diabetics). A caution should also be mentioned. That some forms of prevention could impinge upon the freedom of the old, thus robbing them of one thing they prize, autonomy, in order to obtain something else they value, health, poses an evident dilemma.[65]

I have stressed some of the problems of reducing pain and suffering and attempting to maintain a decent quality of life. They should not be minimized. There will be some acute struggles about how much we can afford for them also, even if of demonstrable value to the health and well-being of the elderly. Their value, however, is that to give them priority over life-extending technologies would signal a change in thinking about the elderly and about the goals of medicine in caring for the elderly. This will be particularly true of the last category of issues I want to mention, that of long-term care, nursing care, and home care. For there is little doubt that the combination of longer life, particularly for those over 85, and accompanying chronic illness poses a special challenge to our ways of caring for the old.

Between 1985 and 2000 the estimate is that the nursing-home population wil increase by 47 percent, from 1.5 to 2.1 million.[66] There will be a corresponding increase in the number and proportion of the elderly requiring some degree of daily assistance and surveillance outside an institution. Both the number of people and the potential costs of adequate care are enormous.[67] The trend has already worked a distorting effect on the Medicaid program, one originally designed to help the poor in general but which now supports more than half of all nursing-home care for the elderly. As a result, only about 40 percent of Medicaid now goes to the non-elderly poor. Medicare provides support for home care only in the form of short-term critical nursing attention in the aftermath of serious health episodes, not long-term home care. Nowhere is the national bias toward acute-care medicine more obvious than in these policies. The lives of the elderly are saved, often at great cost, but there are then scant federal resources to respond to the chronic illness or disability that may be the long-term result. The afflicted can neither remain for long in acute-care facilities, eager to discharge them to reduce costs under DRG pressure, nor easily find community facilities to carry on the needed continuing care.

As have others in recent years, I have become impressed with the philosophy underlying the British system and the way it meets the needs of the old and chronically ill. It has, to begin with, a tacit allocation policy. It emphasizes improving quality of life through primary-care medicine and well-subsidized home care and institutional programs for the elderly rather than life-extending acute-care medicine. An undergirding skepticism toward technology makes that a viable option. That attitude, together with a powerful drive for equity, "explains why most British put a higher value on primary care for the population as a whole than on an abundance of sophisticated technology for the few who may benefit from it."[68] That the British spend a significantly smaller proportion of their GNP (6.2 percent) on health care than Americans (10.8 percent) for an almost identical outcome in health status is itself a good advertisement for the British set of priorities. Infant mortality is 11.5 percent in the United States and 11.1 percent in Great Britain. Life expectancies are, for men, 70.0 years in the U.S. and 70.4 years in Great Britain; and, for women, 77.8 in the U.S. and 76.6 in Great Britain.[69]

No less important is the different orientation toward aging and death that the British system appears to express. They are more readily accepted, and it is understood that the consequences of a desperate struggle to save the lives of the elderly cannot fail to have a distorting consequence for health-care priorities and allocations generally. It is a system that works far better to equalize across the generations the "normal opportunity range" than does our own: it reflects a known and accepted allocation policy that provides incentives for political self-restraint on interest-group demands which our system does not.[70] That our present system fails to meet so many health needs of the elderly, and particularly fails to cope with the emergence of chronic illness as their main burden, would surely suggest the value of a change in priorities.[71] That it could also be an acceptable policy orientation for American elderly is possible, although American individualism and love of technology indicate an important difference in ethos. But the British direction has not been tried and provides the single most promising change in perspective to break the monopoly of high-technology medicine and the endless struggle against aging and death that has been its most willing partner. That the British themselves are tending toward the re-creation of a private health-care system does not disprove the value of their traditional priorities, only the failures of a National Health Service beset by chronic national near-depression conditions.

| Changing Expectations

THE JUSTIFICATION I HAVE PROPOSED for the limitation of life-extending resources for the elderly would make little sense, and be unconscionably harsh, apart from the context of an altered vision of the ends of medicine and of aging. I would reiterate my objection to a rationing scheme that in the name of cost containment would cut back on lifesaving care to the elderly without offering a justification based upon some intrinsic benefit for the elderly themselves and some rich understanding of the place of old age in human life. It is, for instance, economics alone that has led recently to an increase in deductibles under Medicare; and that is not a satisfying rationale. Yet even if the vision of medicine and aging I have sketched might appeal to our detached reason, it would still face the obstacle of a set of expectations that have been tutored to move in a different direction. Could we, for instance, psychologically tolerate the social costs of persuading the elderly to give up some life-extending medical care, or reassure the young about their own old age if they knew they would be faced with a similar denial? Would it not be regressive to use age as a rationing standard since, evidently enough, age criteria would not take account of individual variations among the elderly? Would it not be equally regressive to have the government cease providing life-extending care to the elderly when we could predict, with great certainty, that the wealthy (or the desperate of lesser financial means) would seek to buy that care on the private (or black) market?

Each of those questions turns, in its own way, on our present expectations about what old age is (or at least ought to be). Assuming it is desirable to do so, can those expectations be changed without a sense of severe loss, even tragedy? The only possible answer is that it could not be done easily or quickly and would probably require a generation or more for a new understanding, and new expectations, to take hold. The three objections just stated lend themselves to imagining how that might take place, and I will consider them in turn, using each to build upon the last.

We might begin by recalling two points, one historical and the other contemporary. The first is that a century and more ago, there was no human expectation whatever that medicine could significantly extend individual life or effectively combat the infirmities of old age. It was understood that old age was a part of life relatively brief in duration and was followed by death (and usually a relatively swift death, not the lingering one over a period of years that has now become common—for example, the present average of three years in the case of cancer). That set of facts was not taken to be a fundamental indictment of life itself, nor, so far as I can make out, were old age and death feared any more then than they are now. Hence, we know it is perfectly possible psychologically to have a different, more accepting set of expectations toward aging and death; they are not fixed by human nature. The second point is the near-universal report that, as noted above, it is not aging as such that is feared but the loss of social significance and personal independence with which it has become associated. It is not death in itself that evokes dread so much as a humiliating, oppressive death—either a high-technology death amidst machines and tubes in a modern hospital, or a drawn-out loss of one's faculties in a nursing home, where death seems too long in coming.

Our present expectations about aging and death, it turns out, may not indeed be unambiguously reassuring: we are by no means sure that modern medicine promises us so much better an aging and death, even if some features appear improved and the process begins later. It is not therefore inconceivable that, over time, most people could be persuaded that a different, more limited set of expectations promised to be as satisfying as the present ones. That would be all the more possible if there were a greater assurance than at present that one would live out a full life span, that one's chronic illnesses would be better supported by government programs, and that long-term and home care would be given a more powerful societal backing than is now the case. Though they would face a denial of life-extending medical care beyond a certain age, the old would not necessarily fear their aging any more than they now do, nor would the young—even knowing that life-extending care would be cut off by a certain age—believe their fate to be worse than that of earlier generations. As is the case now, the young could well fear that they would be burdened with the care of parents beyond their economic and emotional resources; but it would be stronger home and institutional care that would relieve that anxiety, not further life-extending care. Expectations could be changed. The future of health care for the aged would be different, but not necessarily, on balance, worse. There would also be the added satisfaction of knowing that because of the limits on research and health-care delivery devoted to life extension for the elderly, a continuing high growth rate for the health-care budget had ceased to be inevitable.

Would we not, however, have bought those developments at a high price, that of systematically excluding the great variation among the aged from consideration? In particular, since it is well known that only a small proportion of the elderly have very high health-care costs and needs, why not focus our rationing efforts on them? By limiting life-extending care to everyone, would we not indiscriminately sweep up many in otherwise fine shape who, with one or two timely medical interventions, might have remaining a number of years of good life? The answer is that we would indeed, in a sense, penalize the latter group; or more precisely, we would not benefit them, despite the fact that they would gain much more from life-extending treatment than those in poor condition. But I see no way to avoid, at some point, a choice that will cause anguish, shorten some lives, and possibly appear unjust.

Recall that the main policy goal would be to assure everyone a chance to live out a natural life span. To deny those in poor health a chance to achieve that goal—particularly in order that others, in better health, might be assisted to live well beyond that point—would be unfair. And I assume that we cannot expect for much longer to pay for both. To deny care to those in poor health would be a denial of a basic good that ought to be available to all and, beyond that, the heaping of additional misery on those whose elderly years are already blighted by illness. But those in good health, by contrast, have already had a natural advantage. Their later years have already been superior years in comparison with their afflicted peers'. A restriction of their care would not be as unfair as a restriction of care for those who have not been so fortunate. With such a shift in priorities, the young could look forward to their old age with less anxiety if assured a vigorous societal commitment to give them a full and natural life span; they would know they would not be abandoned prior to that stage if their health-care costs were too heavy. The use of age as a standard for terminating care would be regressive only if used alone, with no other modifications being made in benefits given the elderly. But it could be the fairest possible means of allocation if combined with an improvement in other benefits. For all would have a guarantee that a minimal and common baseline of accessible health care up through a normal life span would be theirs; only thereafter would differences appear.

By refusing the healthy life-extending care beyond a certain age, we would not, however, be denying them a benefit to which they had a special claim. We would instead be saying that a society in which all were assisted to live out a full life span was more tolerable and humane, both to the old who lived in it and to the young who had it to look forward to in their old age, than our present situation. Since the young cannot know in advance whether they will be in the minority who will require heavy and expensive care in their old age to preserve their lives, their prudence would seem to better justify a health-care system that would support such care through (but not beyond) a full life span than one which did not, even if the latter might extend one's years a bit more beyond that point should one be lucky enough to get that far.[72]

That such a priority system would invite some abuses and create some new problems should not be denied or minimized. A government policy of denying Medicare support for life-extending treatment beyond a certain age would favor those elderly who could afford personally to pay for such care. It could also severely tempt many middle-class families to sacrifice their less-than-ample resources to save the life of a loved one they are not yet ready to relinquish. It would no less tempt physicians, motivated by kindness and a commitment to save life, to evade reimbursement restrictions on life-extending treatment. They could well exploit the often fine, and sometimes indistinguishable, line between the relief of suffering and the extension of life. They could in addition simply manipulate the system in the name of conscience. That is now sometimes done in silent protest against the present DRG Medicare payment system, and was once widely done by many physicians who out of moral conviction falsely certified in the 1960s and earlier that some women needed an abortion because of a threat to their life or mental health.

There would be no simple solution to problems of that kind, and they would occasion sorrow and anguish. As the British and other Europeans have come to learn, many people are not prepared to stay within a health-care system that imposes limitations on care; they are willing to pay personally for private care. That possibility does favor the wealthy and (though the evidence is not yet in) may do harm to the general health-care system. Yet a rigorous effort to enforce egalitarian solutions is a good prescription for an authoritarian society. The benefits of the unfairness (if such it is) of the system I propose would be limited to those beyond a certain age, and precisely because of that advanced age would for most be a limited benefit, to be terminated shortly by death. I do not believe a society would be made morally intolerable by that kind of imbalance.

As for the possible, even likely, resistance of many physicians to tolerate a Medicare system that denied life-extending treatment to patients they felt could benefit from it, only a different understanding of their role would suffice to reduce that resistance. Such an understanding could come only from recognizing, on the one hand, that a continuation of the present attitude toward the open-ended use of medical technology to extend the lives of the aged poses a threat to adequate health care for younger generations; and, on the other, that a plausible (even proper) view of the social ends of medicine and aging provides independent grounds for limiting health care. That recognition will require a major effort to reorient medicine away from its captivity by the modernizing, technology-driven, borderless "medical need" model of care for the aged. It will no less require a parallel reorientation of the general public, who will be as reluctant to give it up as will physicians. Nothing other than a long-extended public debate over many years is likely to suffice to bring about that kind of change. A proposal to limit health care for the aged will be seen as coercive, and a denial of Medicare coverage on grounds of age will seem particularly so. That kind of coercion will be acceptable only if it is understood to be of benefit to the elderly themselves, to the practice of medicine, and to younger age groups. For all those reasons, it probably could not be successfully imposed in the face of widespread opposition. Only a full-scale change in habits, thinking, and attitudes would work to make it morally and socially plausible.

6 | Care of the Elderly Dying

DEATH, WE ARE TOLD, is no longer a hidden subject. That is at best a half-truth. The aged constitute the majority of those who die, some 70 percent, but a specific discussion of their dying is remarkably scant in legal, ethical, and medical writings. That omission is probably not accidental. The modernization of aging induces a sharp separation between aging and death. The latter is often treated as if it had little to do with the former, a kind of accidental conjunction. In medicine, the long-standing tradition of treating patients regardless of their age works against an open discussion, even though many physicians admit it is a consideration in their actual practice. The courts appear to follow a similar tradition. Despite the large number of decisions in recent years bearing on cases of elderly patients, that fact is typically not mentioned, though it is an obvious feature of the cases.

These inhibitions against explicit discussion of the dying elderly doubtless serve a valuable function. They reflect a sensible fear that the aged might be singled out for unfairly discriminatory treatment. They are a way of acknowledging the difficulty of sharply differentiating the medical conditions of the aged from those of other patients. Yet the pervasiveness of backstage debate about the care of the elderly dying among physicians and nurses, jurists and legislators, and the elderly themselves makes it imperative to now deal explicitly with the issue. There are also other reasons for having such a discussion. If, as I have argued, the proper goal of medicine for those who have already lived out a natural life span ought to be the relief of suffering rather than the extension of life, what are the practical implications of that position for the care of the critically ill, or dying, elderly? If the goals of the aging ought to be service to the young and coming generations, what follows for their way of thinking about death? How does the ready availability of technology sway the making of decisions about the dying? I want to start with that last question.

| Medical Technology: A House Divided

ONE OF THE HARDY ILLUSIONS of the past few decades has been the belief that with a few changes in law and attitudes, the dying can be spared excessive medical treatment and be allowed to die a "death with dignity." Yet the termination of treatment seems to remain almost as hard, if not harder, in practice now than in earlier times. That is true with the old as much as with the young. Despite the public debate and soothing words, both the public and physicians remain profoundly ambivalent about stopping the use of life-sustaining medical technologies. It is often and accurately said that the elderly do not want excessive and useless treatment. They greatly fear a death marked by technological oppressiveness, wrapped in a cocoon of tubes and machines. Yet they have also no less come—as we all have—to expect medicine whenever possible to extend their lives as well as alleviate or cure their diseases. These are not logically incompatible impulses, but they can be psychologically at odds.

The few available public-opinion surveys suggest some of that ambivalence. A 1985 Gallup Poll asked the respondents whether they believed that the law should make possible the withholding of life-sustaining medical treatment if that was what a patient wanted. Those 65 and older were significantly *less* in favor of such a law than younger generations: some 68 percent of those 65 and older favored it, 20 percent were opposed, and 12 percent had no opinion. By contrast, the national average for all age groups was 81 percent in favor, 13 percent opposed, and 6 percent with no opinion.[1]

Two fears seem to compete with each other among the elderly: on the one hand, that they will be abandoned or neglected if they become critically ill or begin to die and that few will care about their fate; or, on the other hand, that they will be excessively treated and their lives painfully extended. Death after a long, lingering illness marked by dementia and isolation in the back room of a nursing home similarly competes as a vision of horror with that of death in an intensive-care unit, a dying constantly interrupted by painful and unwanted interventions. There is reason for such fears. Medicine steadily extends to the elderly the use of drugs, surgery, rehabilitation, and other procedures once thought suitable only for younger patients. Ever-more-aggressive technological means are used to extend the life of the elderly. On the whole, the elderly welcome that development—even as they fear some of its consequences. They want, somehow, that most elusive of all goals: a steadily improving medical technology that will relieve their pain and illness while not leading to overtreatment and to a harmful extension of a life.

The difficulty of making accurate prognoses is part of the problem. In all too many cases, technology is used because it is not known that a patient is dying or in irreversible decline. As noted in the previous chapter, the prognosis of a terminal illness is difficult to achieve. Moreover, the problem of prognosis is even greater, a government study concluded, when immediate decisions must be made about initiating treatment. Only for patients who have been fully diagnosed can estimates of survival probability be made. Even then, the probabilities are very likely to be insufficient for guiding decisionmaking about withholding or withdrawing treatment for an individual patient."[2]

The ordinary, almost instinctive, tendency of physicians faced with that uncertainty is then to use technology, to treat with vigor. For his or her part, the patient—who will ordinarily want to live, but may also be fearful of useless overtreatment—will be faced with a no less highly uncertain situation. How sick am I? What are my chances? Both patients and families are likely to have the same inclination as the physician, to treat. Given a normal desire to preserve life and to use available technologies, those impulses of both patients and physicians are understandable. The hard question, therefore, is not why technology is used so much by physicians, or why patients want it no less than doctors. We have to ask instead why it is so hard to *stop* using it, even when patient welfare and plain common sense appear to demand just that.

Technology has sometimes been likened to an addiction, or a force, that takes on a life of its own quite apart from human desires or intentions. That is too fanciful, and a more likely story can be offered. Physicians use medical technology because it generally works. They have been accustomed by their own education and experience to its routine efficacy. It works in part because there is faith in it, a faith strengthened and made credible by constant testing and experimentation. That process of innovation and persistent refinement means that technology is usually always changing while simultaneously more is being learned about its use. As a consequence, different results are achieved at different times, and, ordinarily, improved results. Open-heart surgery works better now than ten years ago, and will be even better next year. Physicians begin with the presumption that most technology will do some good until it is proved otherwise. The fact that a technology failed in one case in the past, or even in many cases, does not prove it will fail in other, similar cases at present or in the future. Medical technology may spring from science, but its use is in great part a matter of art and shifting probabilities. A pervasive ingredient throughout is a psychological imperative to use technology if at all possible. However flawed, however uncertain the outcome, it remains medicine's best, if not only, hope.

We should not see the question of terminating treatment as a sharply focused "yes" or "no" decision to treat vigorously or allow to die, a kind of binary "1" or "0" gateway to life or death. It is more realistically viewed as a continuum in which the odds of effective intervention slowly decline. At age 65, a person (call him Mr. Smith) in otherwise good health who suffers a heart attack will be treated, and the available technology makes the odds of saving him good.[3] Then imagine Mr. Smith being diagnosed for an operable cancer of the colon at age 75, with a 50 percent chance of full recovery. If he is still mentally alert and eager to live, both doctor and patient will most likely choose to go forward with the operation. Imagine still another phase: at 80, he again suffers a heart attack of moderate severity, with the odds of complete recovery if vigorously treated at about 20 percent and partial recovery at about 60 percent. He will probably be treated. Then, at 82, he suffers a moderately severe stroke, one from which his life can most likely be saved but which will almost certainly leave him semiparalyzed and probably only semicompetent thereafter (but amenable to rehabilitation efforts). Thereafter, he gradually declines and suffers a series of other strokes in his mid to late 80s, spending his last years debilitated and demented in a nursing home before dying at 88.

When, in that continuum, was he dying? There is no straight answer to that question, for he was—but for the technology—dying at many points. Each crisis point presented the need to make a choice for or against initiating treatment. A familiar story then unfolded: since physicians generally aim to save life, and since patients ordinarily prefer to live rather than to die, and since at each point there was some realistic hope, treatment was undertaken. The good fight was fought.

Mr. Smith lived on because we expect medicine to continue to devise ever-more-ingenious ways to save our lives. That is why the annual budget of the National Institutes of Health (NIH) has always risen, budget crises or not. Few congressmen can resist the plea to appropriate funds to save lives through medical research. Why should anyone be astonished, much less indignant, that the other message many are trying to deliver—the need to stop treatment—has such a hard time getting through? Unrelenting "wars" against disease are being pursued by thousands of dedicated medical researchers and physicians at the same time that "natural death" legislation is being passed. The former campaigns are much more dedicated and powerful than the latter. We have been told endlessly—and truthfully, with the support of hard data—that more effective emergency care and the improvement of intensive-care units will save additional lives, and that better geriatric rehabilitation services (for which Mr. Smith was an ideal candidate at many points) will help restore the functioning of the lives thus saved. In the meantime, of course, physicians are being exhorted to stop trying so hard to perform technological miracles with those destined—assuming we can know that—to die. The double message is just about perfect, designed for maximum confusion. As a group the elderly dying are to be saved and those diseases which cause death eliminated. As individuals, however, the elderly dying should be allowed to die when it is right to do so and their diseases allowed to run their course.

| Age as a Criterion

COULD WE NOT, HOWEVER, turn to age as a criterion in order to know when to stop, when to say that no more should be done? I want to explore that question in some detail, and one way or another, it will haunt the remainder of this chapter. I say "haunt" because while there are some good reasons to see age as possibly among the criteria for allowing an elderly person to die, it will remain a delicate and difficult task to accomplish well and with moral safety. While I tried, in Chapter 5, to show that age as a policy standard for the denial of some forms of government-subsidized medical care could be defended, how are we to understand the problem at the bedside, at the clinical level?

I want to look first at one great source of confusion: the common failure to distinguish between age as a medical or technical criterion, pertinent to prognosis, and age as a person- or patient-centered criterion. By age as a medical criterion, I mean treating chronological age as if it were the equivalent of other physical characteristics of a patient—that is, as the equivalent of such typical medical indicators as weight, blood pressure, or white-cell count. Just as those characteristics would be reasonable considerations in treating a patient, so also would age if it could be treated as a reliable technical consideration. Age as a person-centered characteristic, by contrast, would be understood as the relevance of a person's history and biography, his situation not as a collection of organs but as a person, to be taken into account when that personal situation could legitimately be considered. I will argue that age as a medical standard should be rejected, while age as a person-centered (what I will call a "biographical") standard can be used.

1• Age as a Medical Standard. The principal use of age as a medical standard would be in prognosis of treatment outcome: how well will an elderly person respond to and benefit from a treatment? In that respect, the main problem in using age as a standard is twofold. It is difficult to disentangle age from a wide range of other conditions that may coexist with old age. Do kidneys fail because a person is old, or simply because of the ravages of a disease that anyone could have, whatever his age? It is no less difficult to distinguish between the general characteristics of the aged as a group and the unique characteristics of any given aged person. The OTA report on aging and life-extending technology medicine notes the difficulties in making the necessary distinctions (which I have reordered slightly to bring out the underlying logic):

(a) increasing age is associated with greater likelihood of physical decline, increased comorbidity, reduced physiological reserve, and cognitive impairment. Clinically, the probability of these decrements increases notably after age 85;[4]

but (b) chronological age turns out to be a poor predictor of the efficacy of a number of life-sustaining technologies (dialysis, nutritional support, resuscitation, mechanical ventilation, and antibiotics);

while (c) efficacy may be lessened for older patients in general;

but (d) improved medical assessment and care could improve that efficacy;

while (e) in any case very little is currently known about differences in treatment outcome that are due to age *per se* and those that are due to increased prevalance or severity of diseases in older ages;

but (f) in some classification systems (for the purposes of, say, admission to an ICU), chronological age functions as a proxy measure for age-associated factors that cannot be easily measured.

I do not cite the OTA material with any intent to amuse. It is a careful set of distinctions based on the best empirical evidence available and makes perfectly clear why age alone is not a good predictor of medical outcome. It also nicely helps explain why physicians can also say that in practice, they do make decisions based on the age of patients—but rarely can give a wholly defensible scientific account of themselves if pressed to do so. The puzzle, I think, is partially explained by the difference between (1) perceiving a patient as a whole person, whose combination, or gestalt, of characteristics makes it evident that he is old rather than young, which makes a difference in his future; and (2) perceiving and medically treating the person part by part, organ by organ. If we look at a person only as a collection of organs, any given characteristic may well be identical with that found in younger persons (some of whom have wrinkled skin, or failing kidneys, or are bald, or have osteoarthritis, for example). Moreover, even if in some cases, with some conditions, we know age to be generally relevant, we may not know where, on a continuum of characteristics of the aged as a group, any particular old person falls in terms of likely medical outcome. For all these reasons, age as a medical criterion is unreliable.

2• *Age as a Biographical Standard.* If we know someone's age, but nothing else about him, what do we know of significance? If the person is old—say, in his 70s (and certainly by his 80s)—we would know that most of his chronological life is in his past rather than his future, would not expect to find him playing football or climbing trees for recreation, might not be surprised to find that most of his friends are older rather than younger people, and might expect him to have two or more physical impairments, minor or major. Certain "age-associated" traits would almost invariably be present. We would already know something of importance about an old person even before we met him: that he stands much nearer the end than the beginning of the continuum that is his life. Yet we still might not know anything of significance about him in other respects: whether he was happy or sad, relatively healthy or unhealthy for his age, lively or dour, optimistic or pessimistic, bright or dull.

Yet what makes him the person he is, and not someone else, is the combination of his age-associated traits and other, more idiosyncratic personal and social traits. That he was very old, with a statistically short life expectancy, would hardly be irrelevant to him as he thought about his life and his future or to the rest of us for many (even if not all) purposes. As Malcolm Cowley has noted, "we start by growing old in other people's eyes. Then slowly we come to share their judgment."[5] We would not make long-range plans with an elderly person the way we might with a younger person, nor would we likely invite him to take charge of strenuous long-term projects, even if he were highly talented. For his part, he would not be likely to undertake a total change in his way of life, such as immigrating to a new country, or undertaking extensive training for a new career. While age alone would not tell us whether he was lively or dour, bright or dull, we would most likely be far more impressed with great physicial vitality in someone that age than in a teenager.

His age would, in other words, surely be a part of our overall understanding of him—not the whole story, but hardly of no consequence either. While many "age-associated" traits will bear on the functioning of an elderly person, age as a biographical trait does not reduce to that. Age encompasses a relationship to time—less time statistically remains for an old person than a young person, and there is more personal history behind him as well. It encompasses a relationship to self-consciousness—life and its prospects will usually be thought about differently. And it encompasses a relationship to the passing of the generations—the old are next in line to pass as individuals. The old know they are old, and so does everyone else. Age is not an incidental trait of a person. Might the combination of age and other characteristics then be allowed to have a bearing on medical treatment, and particularly termination, decisions?

3· The Morality of Age as a Standard. Before attempting to answer that last question, it is necessary to inquire whether it is moral to make the attempt. Some would say no: age as a criterion for the termination of treatment should be ruled out of bounds altogether. A central strand of medical ethics holds that patients should be treated only on the basis of their strict medical needs, and that age should no more influence the way they are treated than should their race, sex, or ethnic background. Dr. Mark Siegler has pointed to one source of the objection, noting that a failure to retain "need-specific

criteria with respect to elderly patients . . . [would] undermine the
traditions of clinical medicine, which are based upon medical need
and patient preferences . . . and [would] undermine the traditions
of our society, which are based upon moral virtues of charity and
compassion."[6] The immediate force of such objections is evident.
While there has been some toleration in the medical-ethics literature
for the idea of rationing by imposing external policy constraints on
physicians, there has been little if any toleration for the idea of
physician rationing at the bedside. Doctors are enjoined by medical
morality to be unstinting advocates for the welfare of their individual
patients and no less enjoined to use medical criteria only—"medical
need"—in making their decisions. Yet it is precisely that tradition
which my approach to limitation of health care for the aged calls into
doubt. The high cost of health care, unrelenting technological developments, and the good of the elderly themselves require that it
be examined afresh.

"Medical need," in the context of constant technological innovation, is inherently elastic and open-ended; as a guide to what is
actually good for patients or what physicians are obliged to give
them, it is highly unreliable. Experienced and conscientious physicians do in fact take age into account in termination decisions, and
always have. Why should we therefore assume that age is not, and
should not be, part of a responsible moral judgment? The problem
in responding to this question is in distinguishing between a medical
and a moral judgment. That an elderly person should be given a
different drug dosage than a younger patient is ordinarily considered
a purely medical judgment. By that statement is meant that if the
aim is proper physical care of the patient in both cases, then different dosages may be indicated to achieve identical outcomes. A judgment of that kind can be based on scientific evidence. But the use
of age as a "medical" indication is ambiguous. If it means that
because of a person's age, medical treatment will be futile, do no
good whatever, then it may properly be called a medical and not a
moral judgment. It is a judgment about medical efficacy only. Yet if
a judgment is also being passed about the worth of the life—that the
treatment is futile not because it will fail technically but because the
life saved is not worth saving because of age—then it has passed into

the moral realm. According to the tradition of medical ethics, judgments about the social worth of a patient's life are unacceptable as grounds for terminating care. That is a solid and necessary tradition; but it does not touch the question of whether age as a standard might be defensible.

There is also another possibility for ambiguity. What is medical "need"? If understood as the needs of a patient's organs, or other physiological systems, treatment may (by ordinary standards) be required; otherwise they will fail. But if "need" is understood to be the needs of the patient as a person, not merely as an assemblage of deficient organs, no clear answer about the requirement of "medical need" may be forthcoming. Then the physician may have to make a moral judgment: will meeting the needs of the patient's organs meet his needs as a whole person? They are not necessarily the same needs. It is not clear which need the tradition invoked by Dr. Siegler has in mind. More than that, the technological possibilities of medicine for organ sustenance, quite apart from overall patient welfare, mean that "medical need" can rarely if ever be kept free of moral evaluation and judgment. The good of organs is always subordinate to the good of the person. There is no such thing as pure "medical need"; it always presupposes some value judgment about the desirability of treatment.

Will it necessarily be the case, as James Childress has suggested, that the use of an age standard would symbolize "abandonment and exclusion from communal care"?[7] That would be likely only if it were widely believed or perceived that an age standard for exclusion from care came into use as a manifestation of society's rejection, denigration, or devaluation of elderly people. It would be a different matter if, instead, it emerged from a prudent effort to find an appropriate balance between the needs of the aged and those of younger generations, and from a conscientious effort to determine, in the face of potentially unlimited technological innovation in care for the aged, where a reasonable limit on care could be set. The "symbolic significance" of an age standard depends not on the mere fact of using age but on the meaning attributed to that fact; context, perceived motive, and articulated rationale determine that symbolic meaning. As I will note more fully at the end of this chapter,

Childress would most likely be right if age were used as a standard in the present situation; but that would not necessarily be the case if its use were transformed so as to be seen as part of an affirmation of old age and not its denigration.

4• Age as a Biographical Standard for Terminating Treatment. How can a combination of age and other characteristics be allowed to have a bearing on the termination of treatment? How, I respond, can it not any longer? If "medical need" is too indeterminate and elastic a concept to be used by itself, then some use of age will be *necessary* to make a judgment about terminating care of the elderly. Since age is an important aspect of the patient as a person, someone who is not just a collection of organs, it falsifies the reality that is part of a person in his fullness to set it aside as irrelevant. Moreover, in addition to being a necessary part of a full and proper medical-moral judgment, age is a valuable and illuminating part, telling us where the patient stands in relation to his own history. There are a large and growing number of elderly who are not imminently dying but who are feeble and declining, often chronically ill, for whom curative medicine has little to offer. That kind of medicine may still be able to do something for failing organs; it can keep them going a bit longer. But it cannot offer the patient as a person any hope of being restored to good health. A different treatment plan should be in order. That person's history has all but come to an end, and medical care needs to encompass that reality, not try to deny it.

More broadly, even if age is not a good prognosticator for treatment efficacy (that is, physiological efficacy), it is a perfectly reasonable standard for treatment reasonableness or desirability. The mere fact that major surgery, or admission to an ICU, or cardiopulmonary resuscitation might save the life of an elderly person does not mean that it ought to be undertaken. A moral judgment must be made about what ultimately serves the patient's welfare. The "age-associated" fact of multiorgan failure with a poor physical prognosis, for instance, might at the least reasonably incline one to spare an elderly patient such vigorous lifesaving efforts. For many people, beginning with the aged themselves, old age is a reason in itself to think about medical care in a different way, whether in forgoing its lifesaving powers when death is clearly imminent, or in forgoing its use even when death may be distant but life has become a blight rather than a blessing. The alternative is not, as some would have it, respect for life but an idolatrous enslavement to technology.

We should want to know not just what chronological age may tell us about the state of a person's body (as a technical criterion), but also what it morally and psychologically signifies for a person to have an old rather than a young body; or what it means for a person to be old rather than young when considering the prospect of painful treatment; or what it signifies to live life as an old person—or as a sick old person—who cannot expect to recapture the vitality of youth, or even of an earlier old age. When considered in those ways, age becomes a category of evaluation in its own right, something reasonable and proper to wonder and worry about. It bears not only on physical characteristics, but on a person's self-understanding, as something intrinsic (with varying degrees of intensity, to be sure) to a person's individuality and life story. The whole person—and it is that whole person who presents himself or herself for treatment—is a person of a certain chronological age: that determines many characteristics, and much of the coloring, of a person's life. That is the importance of the biographical point of view.

| Principles for the Use of Age

How, FROM A BIOGRAPHICAL vantage point, should we formulate age as a criterion for the termination of treatment and make use of it in termination decisions? I will begin by proposing some general background principles for the termination of treatment of the aged, each meant to articulate themes developed earlier:

1• After a person has lived out a natural life span, medical care should no longer be oriented to resisting death. No precise chronological age can readily be set for determining when a natural life span has been achieved—biographies vary—but it would normally be expected by the late 70s or early 80s. While a person's history may not be complete—time is always open-ended—most of it will have been achieved by that stage of life. It will be a full biography, even if more details are still to be added. Death beyond that period is not now, nor should it be, typically considered premature or untimely. Any greater precision than my "late 70s or early 80s" does not at present seem possible, and extended public discussion would be needed to achieve even a rough consensus on the appropriate age range. That discussion would also have to consider whether, for policy purposes, it would be necessary to set an exact age or a range only, and that would pose a classic policy dilemma. Too vague a standard of a "natural life span" would open the way for too great a flexibility of application to be fair or workable, while too specific a standard—one indifferent to the unique features of individual biographies—would preclude prudence and appropriate room for discretion.

Problems of that kind, however difficult, should not be used as an excuse to evade the necessity of setting some kind of age standard, or to conclude that any age standard must necessarily mean denying the value of the elderly. The presumption against resisting death after a natural life span would not in any sense demean those who have lived that long or to suggest that their lives are less valuable than those of younger people. To come to the end of life in old age does not diminish the value of the life; that remains until the very end. This is not a principle, in short, for the comparison of lives. It reflects instead an acceptance of the inevitability of death in general and its acceptability for the individual after a natural life span in particular. Death will then take its proper place as a necessary link in the transition of generations.

2• *Provision of medical care for those who have lived out a natural life span will be limited to the relief of suffering.* Medicine is not in a position to bring meaning and significance to the lives of the old. That only they can do for themselves, with the help of the larger culture. Yet medicine can help promote the physical functioning, the mental alertness, and the emotional stability conducive to this pursuit. These remain valuable goals, even when a natural life span has been attained. The difference at that point is that death should no longer be treated by medicine as an enemy. It may well be, of course, that medical efforts to relieve suffering will frequently have the unintended but foreseeable consequence of extending life expectancy. That is to be expected. A sharp line between relieving suffering and extending life will be on occasion difficult to draw, and under no circumstance would it be acceptable to fail to relieve suffering because of the possibility of life extension. The bias of the principle should be to stop resisting death after a certain age, but not when the price of doing so is unrelievable suffering. At the same time— as the success of the hospice movement proves—it is perfectly possible to relieve suffering while not seeking to extend life.

3• The existence of medical technologies capable of extending the lives of the elderly who have lived out a natural life span creates no presumption whatever that the technologies must be used for that purpose. The uses of technology are always to be subordinated to the appropriate ends of medicine: that is, to the avoidance of premature death and to the relief of suffering. The alternative is slavery to the powers of technology—they, not we, will determine our end. Medicine should in particular resist the tendency to provide to the aged the life-extending capabilities of technologies developed primarily to help younger people avoid premature and untimely death. The use of those technologies should be subordinate to what is good for the elderly as individuals, good for them as members of society, good for them as a link in the passing of the generations, and good for the needs of other age groups.

The three principles detailed above are not so radical as they may first appear. They come close to actually articulating what many elderly express as their fears about aging and death. They indicate a wish that their life not be aggressively extended beyond a point at which they still possess a good degree of physical functioning and mental alertness, a life that has value and meaning for them; they are asking not for more years as such (though some would want just that), but for as many *good* years as possible, and that medical technology be limited in its use to those situations in which it will maintain or restore an adequate quality of life, not sustain and extend a deteriorating life.

The old can, of course, be inconsistent and ambivalent; we all can. Neither they nor the rest of us seem fully to understand how to strain out the essence of a desire only to live a full life from an ordinary fear of death, which leads us to grasp at greater longevity even as we recoil from its undesirable consequences. Neither do we seem to understand how to resist the seductions of a medical technology that promises to give us more life as long as we are not prepared to count the costs. Nor do we grasp how to free ourselves from the mistaken worry that a failure to work hard in favor of longer lives for the elderly will be thought tantamount to ageism or to the systematic neglect and abuse of the elderly.

| Criteria for Terminating Treatment

HOW MIGHT WE PUT the three principles I have suggested into operation? The appropriate moral and legal standards for terminating treatment of competent adult patients provide a natural point of departure, embodying as they do a commonly expressed ideal, a principle of law, and a base point for understanding the rights of persons and patients. What are our rights as we face death or resist further treatment? To put the matter in its most fundamental terms, both the law and common principles of medical ethics accord competent patients the right to determine when they no longer wish to be treated.[8] The patient is to be the ultimate judge of the benefits and the burdens of life-sustaining treatment, and whether the burdens outweigh the benefits. The right to make such judgments rests upon the principle of patient self-determination. This value reflects our society's long-standing ethical tradition of recognizing the unique moral worth of the individual, and of respecting human dignity by granting individuals the right to make choices about their lives and their bodies in ways consonant with their moral and religious beliefs.[9] The principle of self-determination is the moral basis for the legal doctrine of informed consent, which the courts have determined to include the right to informed refusal of treatment. The right of self-determination is, of course, meant to apply to the elderly as much as to any other patients. Neither the courts nor codes of medical ethics make any age distinctions among competent adults in the application of the principles.

I will not elaborate further on this basic right of self-determination. It has been written about well and at length elsewhere.[10] One should note, however, that the full recognition of that right has met many obstacles in practice and still represents an ideal rather than an achieved reality. An underlying obstacle (in addition to simple paternalism) has been the enormous ambivalence toward lifesaving medicine discussed at the beginning of this chapter, experienced at times by both physicians and patients. Another obstacle is the still-common assumption that a desire for the termination of treatment is symptomatic of depression rather than a free, rational choice. Depression is, of course, a real possibility with the critically ill or debilitated elderly as with any other patient. But it is the automatic assumption of depression in the elderly who express a wish to die that is the greatest source of unfairness. Patients' wishes are simply ignored out of a belief that they do not know what they want. The kind of bias that treats the elderly as children is a closely related obstacle. There the assumption is that the elderly person has already left the world of adult competence and has regressed to a childish state. More properly and fairly, only a clear showing that this has happened should be allowed to overcome the patient's judgment.

For at least two decades now, the right of patients to make known their wishes through advance directives has been understood to be a clear implication of the right of self-determination. These advance directives have been formalized in the legal instrument of "living wills" or use of the durable-power-of-attorney method as recognized by the laws of a growing number of states. Under "living will" statutes, patients may state in advance those conditions under which they want treatment terminated, while the durable-power-of-attorney procedure permits the designation of a specific surrogate to make decisions for a person should he or she become incompetent. A continuing problem with "living wills" has been the unwillingness of many physicians to honor them (out of an often misplaced fear of malpractice suits). Stronger efforts to make those documents more binding on health-care workers would be exceedingly helpful. Such problems with the "living will" approach have made a durable-power-of-attorney strategy seem a more effective one, far more likely to achieve fulfillment of the wishes of the patient.

Strikingly absent in most of the discussion and writings on the competent patient, old or young, are considerations of the appropriate and responsible use of the personal freedom and right to terminate treatment. All too often, moral discussion of competent patients begins and ends with a declaration that they have a right to do with their lives as they please and to terminate their treatment when they choose to do so. That is legally true and long a part of our moral tradition. But why should that be thought, as is often the case, to be the end of moral analysis? What should the individual with that right think about? What moral obligations, for instance, might a person have toward his or her own life and future, toward those friends and family members who could be affected by a voluntary decision to forgo treatment, toward the larger community? These can be difficult, even agonizing questions for the elderly, an aspect of trying to sum up and understand one's life as a whole, and of trying in particular to determine when it should appropriately end, when death should no longer be resisted. I do no more than flag the issue here. It is the great missing link in recent discussions of the rights of competent patients: what should be done with the rights once one has them?

The suggestion is occasionally heard that the elderly may have a duty to die, to relieve their family or society of the costs of their care. This is a dangerous notion, a small step away from declaring the old to be useless; it is a natural child of a utilitarian stance toward the elderly and their social value. The very notion of a duty to die embraces the use of the old as means to the ends of others. That cannot be demanded of anyone. To be sure, I have tried to show that the elderly do not have an unlimited claim on health resources. That is a very different matter from asserting a positive duty not to use resources, and a recourse to death as a means to that end.

There is a related question. Is there a right on the part of a competent, but dying, patient to vigorous life-extending treatment when there is little medical reason to think it will be efficacious? That would be a strange claim. A patient has a right only to ask medicine to do that which is compatible with its proper goals. Those goals cannot encompass an effort to extend a life in the face of a wholly bleak medical prognosis; health cannot thereby be promoted. Discretion and sensitivity in the doctor–patient relationship will be required in a refusal to provide wanted though useless treatment. The physician should make clear that he or she cannot provide useless or inappropriate care which will neither do the patient any good nor bring honor to the practice of medicine.

I now turn to terminal decisions for those incompetent elderly who have lived out a full and natural life span and have left no advance directives, when those caring for the patient do not know what the patient wants or values. A surrogate must then decide what serves the good or welfare of the patient. There are a variety of justifiable moral considerations for a surrogate to have treatment terminated and allow death to occur in the case of the incompetent elderly: when their pain and suffering cannot effectively be relieved; when the physical and psychological burdens of their treatment outweigh its benefits; and when a minimally adequate level of functioning of a person in decline can be neither restored nor maintained by further medical treatment. Note that all three of these criteria imply an important presumption: that an otherwise healthy old person, at least until the late 70s or early 80s, ought to be eligible for government-supported lifesaving medical treatment. I am here concerned not with that policy issue but with treatment standards within those boundaries. An immediate question might next arise about these criteria. Could they not apply to persons of any age? Yes, in one sense they could, but in another sense age will add a particular feature to each, and I will try to bring that out as I move along.

1• Inability to Relieve Pain and Suffering. It is customarily said that with sufficient skill and willingness to use whatever dosage is necessary, most pain can now pharmaceutically be relieved. While that may be true, it still makes little sense to maintain for long a life in such a state that only massive and continuous (and ultimately disorienting and consciousness-reducing) dosages can suffice to make it tolerable. The relief of pain, in any case, is not identical to the relief

of suffering. The latter will ordinarily be a manifestation of a realistic hopelessness at the prospect of unending pain, a sense that
one's effective life has come to an end, or that the burden to oneself
of one's illness or frailty is too great to make life worth continuing.
A medicine that can only hold out the prospect of prolonging life in
order to extend, but not relieve, suffering has come to the end of its
resources and purpose. Where age may make a difference in these
cases is that the younger person will still typically not have lived out
a full life span and may have significant goals to accomplish (such as
support of a family) which might justify, even require, the enduring
of pain and suffering. That will not ordinarily be as true of the aged,
and even less so the older they become.

2• Disproportionate Burden of Treatment. Treatment burdens—such
as pain, loss of function, and disfigurement—can sometimes outweigh benefits. There is good evidence that in the case of about 1
in every 6 elderly patients on renal dialysis, treatment is deliberately
stopped and death ensues.[11] The thrice-weekly frequency of the
dialysis combined with its side effects—mental disorientation, fa-
tigue, physical discomfort, depression—make it a treatment whose
personal costs simply seem to some too high. Similarly, surgery is
sometimes refused by the elderly because of the pain it would bring,
the lasting complications or debilities in its aftermath, and the fact
that long survival after the operation is not likely in any case.[12] What
difference does age make, particularly since young people sometimes remove themselves from dialysis and also refuse surgery? In
this as in other burden–benefit cases, age will bring in two additional
considerations: whether a long life can be attained by the burdensome medical procedure; and whether a person still has major life
tasks remaining, such that the burdens seem justified or demanded.
In both cases, age will ordinarily make a difference.

3• Inability to Restore or Maintain Quality of Life. I have said comparatively little about the burden–benefit problem, and about
the relief of suffering, because both shade rapidly into the more
encompassing topic of "quality of life."[13] The term itself is not
felicitous, lacking clear cultural roots and a precise, well-understood
meaning. It invites being stuffed with anything that suits anyone's

fancy. Its only, but redeeming, advantage is that we possess no other term or phrase that adequately does its work. That work is ordinarily twofold: to distinguish the condition of human life from the value of that life (often referred to as the sanctity of life), and between the physical state of a person's body and the larger good of the person as a whole. In that latter sense, it has often been used to distinguish between "vitalism"—the view that life in itself, regardless of its condition, ought to be valued and preserved—and the view that the preservation of life should be determined by the condition of that life. A distinction is often also made between the concept of "quality" as referring to individual worth based on some comparative social standard, and quality based on the inherent health and well-being of a person in comparison with his own potential.[14] A great and justifiable fear is that "quality" as a comparative social standard will be used as a way of denying equality to all human beings and of dismissing some lives as not worthy to be lived.[15] That is a view rightly rejected, in the context of the aged no less than with others.

The idea of the sanctity and value of individual life can have no meaning, however, without encompassing some consideration of quality of life. We value human life, and the personhood that is the crowning glory of that life, because it possesses certain capacities that are the distinguishing marks of human beings, those which separate humans from animals and lend them their power to reflect upon their own condition. To be sure, the possession of those capacities forms a continuum, and there has been a justifiable reluctance to exclude borderline cases from the human community. The evils that result from that tendency were displayed all too murderously under the Nazi regime, which coined the term *"Untermensch"* to designate those determined to be subhuman and dispensable and spoke all too readily of "a life not worth living."[16]

However varied its manifestations, and however faint its expression, the essence of a person's "quality of life" will be the possession of certain potentialities for personhood. The "sanctity of life" has to be the sanctity of personhood, not merely the possession of a body. What are the crucial potentialities for personhood? That is a complex and controversial question, but must at least encompass the capacity to reason, to have emotions, and to enter into relationships with others. Of these three potentialities, the most minimal is the capacity to experience emotions (including the sensation of pain); but it has a special importance in the case of the elderly because it may be, locked behind severe dementia, the only capacity some will have remaining. A person who has lost all of these capacities cannot, in any meaningful way, be called a "person" any longer or be said to have a "biographical life" remaining.[17] But a person who has one of these capacities, even the most minimal one of self-enclosed emotions, can still be said to be a person. At the least, lacking access to such a person's inner life, we should give the benefit of the doubt to those who display evidence of emotions (not possible in the case of a permanent vegetative state).

It is also helpful to distinguish between the loss of a potentiality altogether and the presence of severe physical or emotional impediments that may block its expression. Severe and intractable pain and suffering, or the effects of heavy dosages of medication necessary to relieve the pain, can effectively block a person's capacity to reason and to enter into a relationship with others (and severe pain, while producing emotions, could make it impossible for a person to be at one with himself). A consideration in thinking about the burdens and benefits of a proposed medical procedure would be the likelihood of its effects on those potentialities. We need a way also of understanding the possible impact on the capacities of personhood of the loss of such physical functions as movement, speech, sight or hearing. They can make the realization of the inherent capacities difficult.

My definitions and discussion here have been of necessity general and abstract. Let me now turn to the various modes of terminating treatment to give them more specificity.

| Determining Appropriate Treatment

IN DETERMINING MORALLY APPROPRIATE CARE for the elderly, three major types of considerations should come into play: (1) the physical and mental status of the patient; (2) the levels of possible medical and nursing care; (3) the quality of life of the patient. I want to conduct my analysis on the basis of those considerations, but I want also to divide the analysis into two steps. As a first step, in this chapter, I suggest a number of relatively straightforward ways to make decisions based on quality-of-life standards. My second step, in the next section, will be to look at the problem of uncertainty in making decisions and at the symbolic meaning that some decisions can have. The first step will be relatively devoid of shades and shadows; the second step consists of nothing but.

(I) CLASSIFICATIONS.
    (a) PHYSICAL AND MENTAL STATUS[18]
        (1) Patients with brain death
        (2) Patients in persistent vegetative state
        (3) Patients who are severely demented
        (4) Patients with mild to moderate impairment of competence (or fluctuating competence)
        (5) Severely ill, mentally alert patients
        (6) Physically frail, but not severely ill, mentally alert patients
        (7) Physically vigorous, mentally alert patients

    (b) LEVELS OF CARE
        (1) Emergency lifesaving interventions (example, CPR)
        (2) Intensive care and advanced life support (examples, intensive-care units, respirators)
        (3) General medical care (examples, antibiotics, surgery, cancer chemotherapy, artificial hydration and nutrition)
        (4) General nursing care for comfort and palliation

    (c) QUALITY OF LIFE
        (1) Criteria of quality of life: capacity to think, feel, interact with others

> (2) Impediments to quality: severe pain and
> suffering (or effects of medication
> to relieve them), and any other
> condition that thwarts capacity to
> think, feel, and interact with others

I want to use this classification system for illustrative purposes. It is not meant to explore all possibilities or to exclude other possibilities that might be consistent with the principles I have proposed. A certain suspicion is in order about tidy charts and clean formulas. As one physician observed in a moving article on the care of the debilitated elderly, "it is simply too difficult to define all the varieties of illness, suffering, prognosis, and treatment with sufficient precision for the definitions to be of much help in the actual situations."[19] Implicit in my analysis will be the assumption that Medicare support would be provided only for the level of care indicated.

In the case of a patient who is *brain dead*, no further care of any kind, medical or nursing, is called for. All potential for being a person is irrevocably lost, and only a pronouncement of death is in order. What are we to make, however, of someone in a *persistent vegetative state (pvs)*—that is, a person whose brain stem is still functioning, but whose higher, neocortical brain functions are clinically judged to have ceased? That being has also lost all capacities for personhood, though clinical death has not occurred. Assuming a careful diagnosis (and occasional errors have been reported), all treatment other than minimal nursing care (level 4) should be terminated.[20] There is no reason to believe that even a minimal capacity for emotion exists. Artificial hydration and nutrition may be terminated also; they serve no purpose, and do no honor to the body or the memory of the person who once inhabited that body. Out of the respect due human bodies prior to clinical death, nursing care should be provided. But death should in no way be resisted.

A more complex situation presents itself with a patient who is *severely demented*. On the one hand, he has lost his capacity for reason and usually—but not always—human interaction. On the other hand, there will be no clear ground for believing that the capacity to experience emotions has been lost. Hence, it would be inappropriate to terminate nursing care (level 4) or nutrition and hydration, either artificial or natural. In general, only nursing care at level 4 should be provided, but I would not eliminate artificial hydration and artificial nutrition, because there is sufficient public and medical doubt whether their provision should be classified as a form of nursing and ordinary comfort or as a form of medical care (a dispute I will take up below). The prognosis for relief from severe dementia is poor at best in the old, and in irreversible cases nonexistent. Death need not be aggressively resisted, although general medical care (level 3) would be justified to reduce suffering. Thus, the death of the person, if not the body, is under way and need not be resisted.

Patients with *mild impairment of competence,* or fluctuating competence, meet the criteria of an acceptable quality of life, even if a low one. They can reason (even if poorly), interact with others (even if erratically), and surely experience emotions. Yet if they have lived out a natural life span and death is therefore not to be rejected, advanced life support (level 2) would not morally be required. While life-extending efforts would not be mandatory, general medical care (level 3) to reduce suffering would be. (A grandfather clause would also be needed in some circumstances: life-extending treatment such as insulin for diabetics or dialysis, if begun in early old age, should not be withdrawn in later old age.)

Severely ill, mentally alert patients who have lived out a full life span should receive care that is limited, as a rule, to general nursing care (level 4), unless there is strong reason to believe that general medical care (level 3) would significantly relieve any suffering. Assuming competence, the patient should make his or her own decisions in these cases. Severe illness—particularly if likely to be terminal without aggressive intervention—should preclude emergency lifesaving interventions (level 1) and intensive care and advanced life support (level 2).

Physically frail, mentally alert patients (apart from being able to make their own decisions in any case) would seem appropriate candidates for general medical care (level 3) and, in some cases, emergency care (level 1). If they have lived a full life, however, extended intensive care and advanced life support would be unwarranted at public expense, an unjustifiable effort (unless necessary to reduce suffering) to extend life. Yet with an elderly and frail person whose death might be counted premature, even general medical care (level 3) should take into account the potential impediments to a decent quality that it may entail. In the case of a younger person, it will be more worth risking in order to allow the living out of a natural life span. However, once medical treatment begins to offer rapidly diminishing returns, and serious deterioration is progressing, then strenuous efforts to prolong life seem out of order.

The care of the *physically vigorous elderly person* poses the fewest problems. All levels of care appear appropriate, at least through the first round of illness and disease, and even for those who have lived a natural life span if there is a solid prospect of a few (say, four or five) more years of good life. It is the one category in which an exception to the cessation of Medicare-supported life-extending treatment to those who have lived a full life span would be justified. Only when such a person deteriorates and falls into one of the other categories would it be appropriate (depending upon the circumstances already discussed) to terminate life-extending treatment. But is it not a contradiction to my age criteria—if a person has lived out a natural life span—to say that all forms of treatment are appropriate? I make an exception in this case because I do not think anyone would find it tolerable to allow the healthy person to be denied lifesaving care. One incident, moreover, does not prove that death or precipitous decline is on its way. A second and further incident will be a different matter.

A concluding comment is required on an issue that frequently arises in the use of age as a criterion for terminating treatment. Is it not unfair to have standards of care, and particularly termination standards, that are different for the old than for the young? If it would be reasonable to terminate medical treatment for an elderly person because of a bleak future, should that not be done with the young as well—for instance, in the case of a severely handicapped newborn? We are not forced to draw such conclusions. The elderly have already lived out a full life. They have not been denied (at least because of their age) the opportunities of living a life; and their death deprives them of less than it does a child or young person who has had no such opportunity. Not only does it seem justifiable to work harder, and to take more chances, to save and rehabilitate the life of a sick child, but also to allocate more resources to those conditions which cause premature death than to those which cause death after a long life. This is not, however, to say that the young should be oppressed by medical treatment in order that they might be saved, or that all technological means for extending the life of handicapped or critically ill children should be used. There are many occasions when that would be cruel and termination of treatment would be morally justified. I am only saying that it is proper to have different standards for young and old.

| Choice, Coercion, and Symbols

I HAVE LAID OUT IN A FORMAL WAY a framework for the termination of treatment of the dying elderly (or, if not dying, those for whom termination could be appropriate in the case of a life-threatening condition). In its abstractness it fails, and must necessary fail, to capture the anguish and inherent difficulty such decisions ought to entail; and it is bound to seem too formal and rigid. It should never be an easy matter to allow a person to die, even if reason and morality seem to support us in doing so. Human life is precious. There are, in that respect, three broad and difficult issues raised by the approach I have outlined, each bearing on a problem of both symbolic and literal importance. The first is this: how should we analyze the termination of nutrition and hydration on the one hand, and of antibiotics on the other, and how should we interpret the symbolism of abandonment of the aged that any proposal to deny those forms of care will evoke? That issue will most often arise in the case of those who are no longer competent and are well beyond making their own choices but are not yet dead. The second issue turns on a very different group of persons: those who are still competent and request that they be either killed by their physician as an act of mercy or provided assistance in committing suicide. Should there be a recognized legal right to have such requests respected, and what would be the symbolism for the aged should that happen?

The third issue bears on the implementation of a policy that would deny life-extending treatment to the elderly. As a part of my approach to health care for the aged, they would cease being eligible for government-supported life extension beyond a certain age. How could a plan of that kind be implemented in the face of resistance? What would be possible means of implementation, and what would be the symbolism, of a refusal under various circumstances to provide treatment to the elderly?

The literal importance of these topics will be obvious enough. But why should anyone care about something as vague and insubstantial as their "symbolic" meaning? By calling something "symbolic" I intend to point to the way in which an action, or a policy, signifies our moral stance toward those affected by it. Does it convey, in its larger message and meaning, respect and sensitivity for the aged and their human situation, or indifference, expediency, and insensitivity? Here I am concerned not so much with the expressed purpose and rationale of an action or policy, what its *alleged* intent is, but with the way it is or may be actually interpreted in practice by those affected, or what its actual impact will be. In considering policies for the elderly, we need to ask about their explicit purpose and justification. Those I have already tried to provide. We need no less ask whether those policies will lead the elderly to feel more or less secure, more or less cherished as people, and more or less respected for their social worth. An examination of the possible symbolic meaning of a policy forces us to move beyond its specific rationale to ask about its broader impact; and particularly, to be alert to discrepancies between the explicit and tacit dimensions of policies. It also stimulates a consideration of the possible unintended consequences of policy choices; and it is clear that policies of the kind I am proposing could have many such consequences. We should imaginatively and thoroughly explore what they might be. No other lessons of modern life are so insistent as the harm that can be done by unintended consequences, or the evil that can be done in the name of doing good. My proposals are not exempt from those lessons.

Nutrition and Hydration

THE CESSATION OF FOOD AND WATER, hardly talked about even a decade ago, represents a new historical stage of response to the dying in general, and to the elderly dying in particular.[21] For it is the latter, in their biological tenacity, who can in large and growing numbers live on in a twilight zone, neither actually dead nor quite alive. Yet the stopping of food and water seems to fly in the face of the basic moral imperative to provide at least care and comfort to the dying.[22] At the same time, because it will be the specific cause of death (even if the underlying disease or disability is the ultimate source of an inability to take food and water by ordinary means), it will have the appearance of direct killing rather than mere allowing to die. The widespread repugnance at the idea of denying food and water to the elderly is by no means to be understood as mere sentimentality. It points to some important moral considerations. I want, therefore, to discuss the argument in favor of such a denial in more detail.

The logical crux of the argument in favor of stopping food and water is that (a) if it is considered morally acceptable to stop medical treatment when such treatment can no longer do the patient any significant good, and (b) if the providing of food and water by such artificial means as a tube or intravenous line is a form of medical treatment, then (c) it is as licit to stop the latter as to stop the former; there is no essential difference between them. If it is not wrong to turn off a respirator, which deprives a patient of oxygen and brings about death, why should it be thought wrong to remove a feeding tube?

The logic of that argument is hard to fault, at least within its narrow terms. Then why is it that many, if not most, people—medical personnel no less than lay people—make a sharp distinction between medical care and the provision of nutrition, artificially or not? Could it be a failure to attend to the logic of the situation, which validly erases any significant difference between the two cases?

That is not likely. More to the point is the apparent conflict of two important moral traditions which converge in this issue. One of those traditions is a general moral duty to feed the hungry and give water to the thirsty. The other tradition is one specific to medicine: a duty always to provide care and comfort to patients even if (and particularly if) nothing further of medical value can be done for them; the giving of food and water is a fundamental part of that tradition.[23]

That these two traditions converge in this case is reason enough to explain a spontaneous revulsion at the thought of cutting off food and water. We are being asked to tolerate an action which goes against our deepest moral and social instincts; that is why its importance is often called symbolic (and sometimes dismissed as merely a kind of symbolic or "sentimental utilitarianism"[24]). Some issues are important because they are symbolic. Others are symbolic because they are important—something beyond the immediate issue is at stake. I believe the latter is the case here. At stake is how far and in what ways we are emotionally prepared to go to terminate life for the elderly. That will say something vital about our understanding of our obligations toward them and the respect owed them. Are we, in brief, to say that the tradition of always caring, even if nothing more can be done, is to give way to something else, a more certain guaranteeing of death? Perhaps all the necessary moral distinctions can be made, and perhaps we can avoid abuse, and perhaps care in general will not suffer. Perhaps, perhaps.

Yet we should know that it is no light matter, or merely symbolic in a trivial sense, to begin tampering with traditions such as continuance of food and water, based on considerable experience. They were cultivated to provide as solid a fortress as morality can offer against a human propensity—seen time and again with the elderly— to neglect, abuse, or kill the powerless, the burdensome, and the inconvenient. Given the need to reduce health-care costs—especially long-term nursing care, which will be the usual site of feeding-cessation decisions—and the fact that the oldest old often have no one to speak in their behalf, there is every reason to hesitate, even to be suspicious. Moreover, it is one thing to make an occasional exception to the general rule to provide food and water as part of minimal nursing care (level 4)—particularly when, as happens occasionally, this provision is a direct cause of pain and discomfort—and still another to make it a routine way to help death along.

I am hesitant about the latter development because it will require the undoing of many valuable ingrained moral habits and ways of thinking. The baneful consequences of this undoing would be a coarsening of sensibilities toward the elderly dying and critically ill who are not in pain or obviously suffering, a psychological distancing and deliberate numbing to facilitate termination of hydration and nutrition, and a blurring of the line between caring for the dying (while not standing in the way of their death) and hastening their dying for our benefit rather than theirs. There is no way of demonstrating that that will actually happen, and a reflexive invocation of a "slippery slope" argument serves little purpose; for all of morality requires that we make distinctions, and every distinction is a slippery slope to somewhere. But the fact that vigorous efforts would have to be made—by intensive desensitization efforts—to overcome the common repugnance at doing such a thing could psychologically begin to make those consequences possible.

That some elderly would benefit from the withholding of food and water would seem undeniable. This would be true at least for that small number of competent, alert patients whose dying is being prolonged, perhaps painfully so, by nutrition and hydration. For those who are incompetent, if a solid case can be made that it is morally acceptable to stop medicial treatment on the ground that it is useless or burdensome, it should be no more difficult to make the same case for stopping artificially provided food and water. Yet perhaps we should pause at this point. Are the elderly as a group no different from any other age group? There is at least one basic reason to think they are different: they are the only age group for whom decline and death are inevitable. The paradoxical reason, therefore, why we should worry about a routine stopping of nutrition and hydration in the case of the elderly as a group is that they are the prime candidates for and potential objectives of such a treatment policy.

Just which patients in particular are at issue here? The occasional patient who persists in living long after medical treatment is stopped would hardly be likely to occasion a major debate about the withholding of food and water. This is a debate, I suggest, primarily about the way we are in the future to think about the care of the frail and demented elderly. It is their frequently pitiful condition that will most commonly press the question of stopping food and water; it is that same condition which should make us hesitate. Should we allow our fears about abuse to overshadow the possible benefits to individual old people, we may fail to respect their rights and dignity. Should we think only about individual benefits, we may naively overlook the wedge of potential abuse we have introduced. The fact that most severely debilitated and demented frail elders have long since lost all beauty, charm, and human grace—indeed, have lost most of what made them distinctive individuals save for a body that refuses to stop functioning—makes them all the more vulnerable. They can be a sharp reminder of our own coming frailty and mortality; and they can cost an enormous amount of money to maintain over many months or years.

How are we to find the right moral course? The route of greatest moral safety—a kind of defensive vitalism—would be to require the provision of artificial hydration and nutrition whatever the circumstances. That would be hard to justify, especially if we have already accepted the idea that artificial feeding is inherently no different from medical care. Even if we think there is a difference, and that food and water are not to be likened to medical care at all, there are still those circumstances, perhaps rare, when food and water painfully extend a dying life. Only a rigid and impersonal dedication to unalterable moral principles (a kind of insensitivity in itself) would lead to those patients' being asked to bear their suffering lest its relief should open the way for abuse in other cases. The opposite route would be to say, simply, that whenever medical treatment can morally be stopped, artificially provided food and water can also be stopped. Yet that option would lead the way to—in fact, would require—a systematic retraining of health-care workers to suppress their ingrained repugnance at withholding food and water.[25] It could of course be no less horrifying for family members.

Neither of those tidy, incisive answers is likely to have a strong future. We will more likely be left with those considerations which are complex, requiring delicate distinctions; and with those answers which will make most decisions hard, uncomfortable, and uncertain. The first distinction of importance is between the frail elderly who are imminently dying and those who are not. The cessation of painful or otherwise burdensome artificial nutrition and hydration for that class of patients is the easiest to justify as part of a broader acceptance of the moral legitimacy of terminating useless or burdensome treatment of the dying. Artificial feeding is a medical procedure. What about those who are not dying but are irreversibly comatose? Again, if it would be justifiable to stop medical treatment, it would appear equally justifiable to stop artificially supplying food and water. Neither provides any genuine benefit to the patient; there is no meaningful life present. It is a mere body only, not an embodied person.

How about an elderly person who is wholly and most likely irreversibly demented, but not obviously in danger of imminent death or a totally vegetative state? Unless there is some good reason to believe that the patient had at one time expressly stated that he or she would not want to be kept alive under those circumstances, or that that could reasonably be inferred from more indirect evidence, I see no justification, under those conditions, for withholding food and water. We cannot know what, if anything, is going on in the mind of such a person; but neither can we infer that *all* human capacities have been lost, including the experiencing of emotions. Clearly they have not all been lost, for the patient will babble and show other signs of feeling. We cannot, therefore, speak with any certainty about what benefits such a person, much less confidently judge that life itself is a burden. That uncertainty should be enough to make us hesitate. Combined with the significant potential for abuse in such cases—someone else's welfare, not that of the patient, coming to be made the test—the line against termination should be drawn here, a very firm and sharp line.

There is a possible price to be paid for drawing the line at this point. There may be some patients who, deep within their inaccessible minds, want to die and resent the fact that those who have power over them do not allow that to happen. Those demented patients who constantly pull out feeding tubes are giving a clear signal. They should not be force-fed. Others, unable to so act, may feel the same, but we will never know. They may be saved against their (unknown) will only to die a more unpleasant death at a later time, for which we would then bear responsibility.

The maintenance of still others might result in a financial burden to society that would directly deprive others of resources they need. It would not be pleasant to look straight in the face at statistics showing that the young must forgo what they need to enable those barely still in the human community to continue lives of highly doubtful meaning or personal benefit. Nonetheless, that is a risk worth running. We need to ask about the social burdens and benefits of standing policies that would allow, and perhaps in the future institutionalize, the routine stopping of food and water. What kind of society would that tend to produce, what kind of medical practice and medical practitioners, and what kinds of policies and attitudes toward the elderly? We do not yet know the answers to questions of that kind, and that is a good enough reason to move slowly and carefully, testing each move not just by rule and principle, but also by the fruit of experience.

Age alone, I note finally, would never be a sufficient reason to terminate artificially provided food and water. For one thing, there is too much public uncertainty about the symbolic meaning of food and water to justify stopping their use with the elderly; the sickest among them are the most powerless. That symbol of basic care should be allowed to remain, even in the face of doubt. For another, since artificial nutrition and hydration are, for many, morally placed in the realm of caring rather than curing, there is no good reason to mount an assault on that belief, even if in the eyes of others it is incorrect. It is not evident that any serious harm is done the individual or the community by maintenance of artificially provided food and water if it causes no pain to do so, and if there is no reason to believe the patient had ever expressed opposition to that form of care. That is sufficient justification to continue it in the borderline instances.

I began this discussion by noting that it is the treatment of the frail and demented elderly that is ultimately at stake in the debate over food and water. Are the reasons I have given for hesitating to stop artificially provided nutrition and hydration equally valid in the case of providing life-sustaining antibiotics or antimicrobials? That is a crucial question because it is those simple technologies, not intensive-care units or open-heart surgery, which keep large numbers of irreversibly demented or severely ill but not terminal old people alive. I do not think the two situations are the same. While they can be relatively inexpensive and a routine part of ordinary care, antibiotics are clearly medical in nature and, in many cases (such as pneumonia), can be every bit as efficacious in extending life as time spent in an intensive-care unit. Their low cost and their simplicity of application are thus beside the point: if there are good reasons to terminate medical treatment of a dying elderly person— or not to resist the onset of a potentially fatal illness—there is no reason to exclude antibiotics from the roster of such treatments.

What about those elderly who are not dying? The same considerations apply. If a patient's quality of life, his potentiality for personhood, has been seriously enough compromised that even general medical care (level 3) is not morally required, then once again the fact that the antibiotics are inexpensive and simple to provide is irrelevant. To put this another way: if we should rightly hesitate to subject the severely demented elderly patient who has lived a full, natural life span to aggressive life-extending treatment in an ICU, or subject the patient to elaborate cancer surgery, we would be equally justified to withhold antibiotics. Pneumonia should be allowed to become, once again, "the old man's friend."

| Euthanasia and Assisted Suicide

THERE ARE MANY TROUBLING FEATURES about the regular or routine cessation of hydration and nutrition for the elderly, even if justifiable in some circumstances. By contrast, the initial attractions of legalized mercy killing (positive euthanasia) and assisted suicide for the elderly are many. They would serve as a capstone of the proclaimed right of the elderly to control their living and their dying. If their illness and decline could not be controlled, at least their death could be. Mercy killing and assisted suicide would no less serve as a readily available, voluntary alternative to the fear of helplessness and dependence that is one of the great threats of old age and an extended dying. The elderly who chose that option could have the assurance of not burdening others. They would also allow in some cases the averting of a painful or terrifying or humiliating death. So many, indeed, are the attractions of euthanasisa and assisted suicide that it might seem obvious for me to commend them as part of a policy of limiting life extension for the elderly.

My conclusion is exactly the opposite: a sanctioning of mercy killing and assisted suicide for the elderly would offer them little practical help and would serve as a threatening symbol of devaluation of old age. I want to be clear about my argument here. I will not develop a full account of the problem of euthanasia and assisted suicide; that is beyond the scope of this book (though I will say that I oppose it). I want only to consider a much narrower question: Would a policy of euthanasia and assisted suicide be of special benefit for the elderly and be more readily justified for the elderly than for younger age groups? It is in answer to that question that I want to say no.

The traditional basis for a claimed right to euthanasia (and a similar argument applies to assisted suicide) is that individuals have absolute dominion over their own bodies. If their death will not do harm to others, then they have a right to will their own death and to seek the means necessary to achieve it.[26] I will pass over here some special and obvious moral and legal problems about the use of third parties to help a person accomplish that end. Assuming that those problems can be handled, what might the special claim of the elderly be? A number of commentators have responded to that question. For Doris Portwood, author of *Common Sense Suicide*, the reason is that "hundreds of thousands end their lives in baffled misery in the near imprisonment of nursing home or hospital. Others are alone. . . . Few would choose any of the common fates of the ailing elderly."[27] For Derek Humphry and Ann Wickett, cofounders of The Hemlock Society, the high costs of care for the elderly, the lack of control many have in their dying, and the likelihood of abuse at the hands of a system bent on controlling costs all point to the need for greater patient control; and euthanasia provides the best and most effective means of control.[28] For Robert S. Morison, the growing range of problems in caring for the old point to the need to "encourage the growing change in attitude toward the individual's right and capacity to select the time, place, and circumstance of one's own last thing."[29] Various public-opinion polls have been cited to support the perception of such a change of attitude.[30] The historical support of Roman stoicism, assorted tribal customs, and other precedents are often cited. That the majority of recent (and more frequent than earlier) "mercy killing" cases in the United States involved elderly patients is sometimes mentioned to suggest greater pressures on the elderly than in previous times.[31]

These are not persuasive claims. Anyone at whatever age suffering from a terrible illness, whether terminal or not, will be greatly burdened; all will seek relief. There is nothing unique to the aged in the desire to have surcease from pain, in the fear of an extended dying, or in the wish not to burden others. Old age in and of itself seems to offer no greater reason for despair or distress than any other age. Younger people with similar conditions may actually have the more depressing prospect—even more years of suffering than the old to which to look forward. That life may hold out few if any future prospects for some elderly persons is true enough, but a young person faced with decline and death does not have good prospects either. In many of the recent "mercy killing" cases, it seems to have been as much the pressure upon the caretaker as sympathy for the person killed that was behind the death, a point recognized by Humphry and Wickett.[32] More supportive help for the caretaker might have averted the death. While the suicide rate for the old is higher than that for younger people, it has not increased significantly in recent years, and researchers on suicide do not attribute it to age (or the illness that may accompany it). Despite the fact that older women are poorer, and live longer lives, some three-quarters of suicides among the elderly are men, and 60 percent of those are among men living alone. Lifelong problems, psychiatric or social, seem to offer a more promising explanation of suicide among the elderly.[33] If a case can be made for a "rational suicide," there is no special reason to think that old age by itself automatically qualifies. Here is a place where the diversity of the aged is especially manifest: they react to the reality of pain, chronic illness, and impending death with as wide a range of responses as any other age group.

Those matters are, however, open to debate and different interpretations. It is sufficient in this context simply to recognize that there is no straight and inevitable line between old age, even very sick old age, and a desire for an assisted death. Were euthanasia and assisted suicide to be legalized, would there be a large and hitherto restrained group of elderly eager to take advantage of the new opportunity? There is no evidence to suggest that there would be, in either this country or in any other. But even if there might be some, what larger significance might the elderly in general draw from the new situation? It would be perfectly plausible for them to interpret it as the granting of a new freedom. It would be no less plausible for them to interpret it as a societal concession to the view that old age can have no meaning and significance if accompanied by decline, pain, and despair. It would be to come close to saying officially that old age can be empty and pointless and that society must give up on elderly people. For the young it could convey the message that pain is not to be endured, that community cannot be found for many of the old, and that a life not marked by good health, by hope and vitality, is not a life worth living.

Both the modernizing and prolife positions are likely to abet a movement toward euthanasia, but for reasons neither of them may suspect. In the case of the modernizers of old age, it is decline and death that cannot be tolerated; they are the enemies. Only survival has meaning and value. Only physical and psychological vitality and an aping of the young or middle-aged can provide social significance. The embracing of euthanasia indirectly concedes something about old age that modernizers would prefer remain in the shadows but that is implicit in their stance: it has no value save for the possibility of transcending its limitations. If that cannot be done—which at present it cannot—then euthanasia offers an attractive escape. A prolife stance may have a similar outcome. If it is successful in its attempts to oppose any cessation of treatment save for the most hopeless cases, it would be likely to keep alive, and in despair, many who would wish for more benign deaths. They would find a policy of legalized euthanasia and assisted suicide a special relief, one that would not be required but for prolife intransigence and the implicit unwillingness (despite denials) of its following to accept death.

What do we as a society want to say about the elderly and their lives? If one believes that the old should not be rejected, that old age is worthy of respect, that the old have as valid a social place as any other age group, and that the old are as diverse in their temperaments and outlooks as any other age group, an endorsement of a special need for euthanasisa for the old seems to belie all those commitments. It would be a way of legitimizing the view that old age is a special time of lost hopes, empty futures, and personal pointlessness. Alternatively, if it is believed that old age can have a special value, that it can—with the right cultural, economic, and political support—be a time of meaning and significance, then one will not embrace euthanasia as a special solution for the problem of old age, either for the aged as individuals or for the aged as a group. It would convey precisely the wrong symbolism. To sanction euthanasia as a special benefit for the aged would signal a direct contradiction to an effort to give meaning and significance to old age.

| Choice and Coercion

I HAVE SAVED FOR LAST a confrontation with the possible symbolic meaning of my proposal that life-extending medical care be denied to some elderly people under some circumstances as a part of government health-care policy. A skeptic might well note that a policy of that kind could appear a most harsh rejection of the sick and feeble old, as mean-spirited a symbol of societal devaluation of the elderly as could be imagined. I fully agree about that possibility under the present circumstances. If that kind of policy were instituted without a change in our present understanding of old age and death—without a reformulation of the ends of medicine and aging—

it could do great harm and convey damaging messages to the old. *Cessation of life-extending treatment for the aged as a matter of social policy can be morally acceptable only within a context that accords meaning and significance to the lives of the individual aged and recognizes the positive virtues of the passing of the generations.* Yet even if the general coherence of my approach is recognized—particularly the necessary inseparability of a policy limiting care and a highly positive vision of old age—there remain some troubling details, many of which carry with them the possibility of a potent negative symbolism and difficult policy decisions.

Let us imagine that the idea of limiting life-extending health care for the elderly under conditions roughly similar to those I have sketched has been accepted as a matter of public policy. Thereafter, to implement the policy, Medicare benefits would be denied to some elderly people in ways consistent with the policy; and some would die as a direct consequence. But what about those elderly or their families who resisted such a policy? Three political responses are imaginable. The first would be to do nothing to deter those elderly or their families from paying for life-extending care out of their own pockets; it would simply be that they could not claim Medicare or other forms of government support. If that policy were paralleled by a set of attitudes and an ethos among physicians supportive of providing such private care, at least some number of elderly would probably be able to afford it. Another imaginable strategy might join a denial of Medicare benefits with a widespread, though not legally mandated, stance among physicians that not just government policy, but the proper goals of medicine would militate against even the private provision of care. Even if there were some dissenters who would provide the desired treatment, physicians on the whole would consider it harmful to medicine and society to provide care of that kind. The harshest imaginable tactic would be one that legally forbade physicians to provide some forms of life-extending care even if they could be paid for privately.

Each of those possible means of policy implementation carries both practical and symbolic problems. To make life-extending care available only to those who could pay for it would not necessarily mean that only the rich or affluent would benefit. It could and no doubt would invite desperate efforts to raise the needed money among those of modest means; they could spend themselves into impoverishment. It might well trouble the conscience of those physicians who took that kind of private money to save lives. The negative symbolism of a society and a medicine that denied life-saving care to those too poor to pay for it need not be elaborated upon. It could be potentially troubling at the least, and scandalous if widespread. Would it make a difference if most physicians supported the rationale for a denial of life-extending care to some elderly patients and thus refused to treat them even if supported privately? That might bring some relief if only because it would signify a serious commitment to the moral reasoning behind the government policy; it would bespeak a larger social consensus. At the same time, the likely prospect that some desperate elderly patients or their families would have to go to additional trouble to seek out those physicians who rejected the views of the majority of their colleagues might be less than edifying. It could have about it a furtive and illicit aura even if not actually illicit in itself.

To make such care explicitly unlawful would pose another set of problems. Efforts to outlaw those goods or items which many people eagerly want, and often feel morally entitled to, are usually beset with enforcement problems and usually breed additional crime as an offshoot (think of the efforts to prohibit the use of alcohol in the 1920s, abortion through the 1960s, or, more recently, pornography and drugs). A lucrative black market in the saving of life among the elderly is all too plausible a scenario under any outright prohibition scheme. That is not an attractive possibility, and symbolically it is highly distasteful—people being forced to break the law in order to stay alive.

I am trying here to look at my proposal to limit life-extending care with as realistic and candid an eye as possible, giving it not the benefit of doubt but the solvent of skepticism. It is not an idea to be accepted casually, without thought being given to its practical implications. Even if it came to make sense to people as a way of long-range thinking about health care for the elderly, it would still pose some extraordinarily difficult implementation problems. There would, at a minimum, have to be a strong social consensus in its favor to lead legislators and others to be willing to tackle the practical problems (analogous, for example, to the kind of consensus that forged the federal tax-reform act of 1986, or the 1983 Medicare reform effort). The old would have to understand that the intent behind a policy of limiting care would be the welfare of the elderly and of younger generations, and that it was affirmative toward old age and not simply mean-spirited. The young would have to understand that while their own eventual old age would be marked by limits of a kind not earlier experienced by the elderly, they would on balance have a better old age than was earlier the case.

Both the young and old, that is, would have to understand that the combination of constant technological progress and a growing proportion of elderly had conspired to force a new reckoning with old age and its meaning. They would have to respect the fact that a policy of limitation grew out of a long period of societal self-reflection, one that produced a heightened sense of responsibility to future generations, a serious reconsideration of the appropriate goals of medicine and old age, and a fresh acceptance of some ancient wisdom: that old age and death are inevitable and not inherently evil. Only the symbolism of a serious societal self-reflection which led to an outcome of that kind could serve to override the harsh symbolism, of a kind outlined above, that would be implicit in working through the details of a denial of that medical treatment which saves lives. I do not deny the complexity of that task. Neither do I see an easier alternative. The present course embodies the public pretense that there is at present no serious, or at least unmanageable, problem of actual and escalating rationing. The form that rationing is taking, which is simply to make the elderly pay for an increasing share of their care, is neither fair, open, nor forward-looking. Rationing by age is not desirable in many respects, but it is far more desirable than any other solution that has been offered. But then, no long-term solutions have been offered.

7 | Old Age in New Times

AT THE END of his important 1975 book *Why Survive?: Being Old in America*, Robert N. Butler, soon to become the first director of the new National Institute of Aging, quotes the ancient Greek poet Pindar: "Do not yearn after immortality. But exhaust the limits of the possible." That quotation is immediately followed by some concluding reflections by Dr. Butler: "What can be done about humankind's uneasy knowledge that life is brief and death inevitable? There is no way to avoid our ultimate destiny. But we can struggle to give each human the chance to be born safely, to be loved and cared for in childhood, to taste everything the life cycle has to offer, including adolescence, middle age, perhaps parenthood and certainly a secure old age; to learn to balance love and sex and aggression in a way that is satisfying to the person and those around him; to push outward without a sense of limits; to explore the possibilities of human existence through the senses, intelligence and creativity; and most of all, to be healthy enough to enjoy the love of others and a love for oneself. After one has lived a life of meaning, death may lose much of its terror. For what we fear most is not really death but a meaningless and absurd life."[1]

That is a wonderful passage, as moving now as it was when first published in 1975. Yet there is a problem in it. Notice that Dr.

Butler first quotes Pindar, who in a few brief words says we should "exhaust the limits of the possible." Only a few sentences later, Butler says that we should "push outward without a sense of limits." He does not explain what he means by that phrase, and the apparent contradiction between it and the Pindar quotation is left standing as the book ends. The contradiction is not simply Dr. Butler's. We all share it. We know that life has limits, that death lies at the end of old age. We have just not as a society been prepared to accept those hard truths without a struggle: without first—through the agency of medicine—stretching those limits as if they were not there; and then—through the redefinition of old age as an open frontier and not a closed boundary—all but denying there must be limits. Pindar had it right the first time.

That the contradiction has gone unacknowledged is perhaps understandable. Dr. Butler's book was powerfully influential because it articulated an insight that had been slow to sink in, even into the 1970s: despite the obvious demographic fact that a larger number and proportion of people were living into old age, far too many still lived in poverty, in terrible housing, denied the right to work, too often condemned to terrible nursing homes, to poor medical care, to gross and subtle forms of victimization—and assumed, all the while, to be universally frail, senile, and burdensome. He could speak plausibly of "the tragedy of old age in America," of "growing old absurd" (the titles of his first and last chapters), and, most memorably, of "ageism," which he had earlier (in 1968) defined as "a process of systematic stereotyping of and discrimination against people because they are old, just as racism and sexism accomplish this with skin color and gender."[2] Out of ageism came the "myths" of an inflexible progression of aging, indifferent to individual variations, of unproductivity, of disengagement, of inflexibility, of senility, and of serenity.[3] How were ageism and the myths it nourished, on the one hand, and the actual deprivations and poverty of the aged, on the other, to be combated? By a vigorous program of social reform, by medical research, by public education, and by an organized and politically active cadre of the elderly themselves.

That was a potent and attractive agenda, undeniably valid in its analysis of the troubled, often horrible lot of the elderly, and full of good political sense in its strategy to do something about it. Now, well over a decade later, there is still much to be done on the original agenda. Ageism has not been banished, even if it has been attenuated. Many hundreds of thousands of old people still live in poverty, especially that fastest-growing group of all, those over 85. The medical needs of the elderly are still enormous.

Since there is so much still to be done, how can I seriously propose that a new, altered agenda is necessary? For three reasons: first, because what was a sensible approach for an immediate crisis—a politically energized reform movement stressing abuses and unmet basic needs—is not necessarily the best strategy for the long run; second, because even a decade ago, hardly anyone had a full sense of how penetrating the demographic, medical, and economic changes would and could be—longer lives, rising chronic illness, escalating costs; and third, because there was at the heart of the antiageist reform movement a fundamental contradiction and incoherence—medical progress without limits for human beings whose nature it is to age and die—one that could come into full sight only as some of the earlier economic and social crises had been dealt with and the long-term panorama began to make its outlines visible.

A new way is needed, but not the one that is being pursued, an uninhibited effort to make of old age a new way of life. Its deep inconsistencies, incoherences, and contradictions have now made themselves known; and they in turn rest upon some deeper incoherences within the underlying culture. While it has been an economic crisis, or near-crisis, that forced a sharper look at age and health policy, it is possible that we could muddle through that situation—squeezing, cutting, nibbling, excising, cost-containing, juggling, and scrounging—for some years to come, paying a high price in equity and adequacy of care to be sure, but somehow getting by. A preferable course would to be use the present occasion to ask some more fundamental questions about what we ought to be after. One more proposal for a shift in financing the Medicare Trust Fund, or for a change in codeductibles, or for expanded and improved HMOs—while helpful enough in their own ways and congenial to the incrementalist modes of ordinary politics—will not do the kind of job now necessary, that of asking what we want to make of medicine and aging.

We need to start from the bottom up, with a different vision of the future of aging, medicine, and health care than the one bequeathed us by the reform movement of the 1960s and 1970s. But what might we get if we replaced the common notion of refusing to accept limits with Pindar's more ancient vision of exploring the limits of the possible?

We would, as the necessary first step, refuse to allow technology to set the agenda of the "possible," as if what is technologically feasible were humanly good. Our goals for medicine and aging would set those limits, based not on what technology could do, but on what we think it *ought* to do in light of wise human ends. We would also learn to distinguish between tragedy, outrage, and sadness. It is a tragedy when life ends prematurely even though it is possible to save that life, and when old age is full of burdens even though resources are available to relieve them. It is an outrage when, through selfishness, discrimination, or culpable indifference, the elderly are denied what they need and deserve. But it is only a sadness, an ineradicable part of life itself, when after a long and full life a person ages and dies in a society that has cherished and supported that person through the various stages of life. It is wise to want to banish the tragedy and outrage, but not the sadness.

We would try to discover how to have a common moral dialogue about the ends of medicine and aging—not leaving each of us up to his or her own autonomous devices for coping with such fundamental human and social questions. We would talk with greater depth about death and how we ought to understand and face it—not just leaving ourselves free to devise an autonomous death of our own choosing. We would encourage the generations to talk together to understand their mutual responsibilities—not leaving them, as we do now, to seek their own interests and to fend for themselves.

| Filling the Gaps

NONE OF WHAT I HAVE PROPOSED is likely to be possible or even make much sense unless some additional problems are considered as well. Discerning the proper ends of medicine and of aging must be worked

out in a larger moral and social context. Four questions are particularly salient in that context: How might we best think of the mutual obligations and equitable relationships of the generations to
each other? What is the place of the pursuit of health among the
other goods and needs of society? How does the care of the elderly
relate to the future of the Medicare program? How might we best
interpret the agendas of modernizing and prolife groups on health
care and the elderly? I can do no more than signal the centrality of
those topics for the public debate on the care of the elderly, but it
is important to do at least that much.

1• The Mutual Obligation of the Generations. In 1935, at the advent
of the Social Security system, the elderly were one of the poorest of
all social groups. The program led over the next few decades to a
remarkable change in the lot of the elderly. Nothing comparable,
however, was developed for another needy group, that of children
living in families of poverty. Especially during the 1980s, as the
situation of the elderly has improved, social support for health and
other forms of care for the young has declined. By the mid-1980s,
the consequence of this imbalance had become obvious. In 1960, 35
percent of the elderly were below the poverty line, and 26.5 percent
of children. But by 1983, only 12 to 14 percent of the elderly were
in that situation, while the proportion of children living in poverty
had grown to 21.7 percent. The situation was even worse for minority groups. Elderly blacks had 36.3 percent of their group living
in poverty, while some 46.3 percent of black children were in that
condition. In 1970, poverty among children under 14 was 37 percent
less than poverty among the elderly. But by 1982, the incidence of
poverty among children was 56 percent greater than among the
elderly.[4] Children receive one-sixth as much in federal expenditures
as the elderly.

When Samuel Preston in his 1984 presidential address to the
Population Association of America called attention to these and other
discrepancies, he set afoot a debate that still remains unresolved.
"There is surely," he wrote, "something to be said for a system in
which things get better as we pass through life rather than worse.
The great leveling off of age curves of psychological distress, suicide

and income in the past two decades might simply reflect the fact that we have decided in some fundamental sense that we don't want to face futures that become continually bleaker. But let's be clear that the transfers from the working-age population to the elderly are also transfers away from children, since the working ages bear far more responsibility for child rearing than do the elderly."[5] Preston's article had an immediate impact. The formation shortly thereafter of Americans for Generational Equity (AGE), devoted to promoting debate on, among other topics, the burden to future generations, but particularly the Baby Boom generation, of "our major social insurance programs,"[6] signaled the outburst of a struggle over "intergenerational equity" that still continues.

The most detailed and compelling responses to Preston's address, and to the formation of AGE, were the 1986 publications of the American Gerontological Society *The Common Stake* and *Ties That Bind*.[7] Part of this rebuttal was simply to urge that the idea of intergenerational competition reflected an unduly pessimistic and divisive view of America's future. By adopting a "fixed pie" perspective, the age-competition viewpoint mistakenly assumed that resources could not be enlarged to meet the needs of both young and old, or that new policies and new ways of allocating the federal budget could not be devised. It was, therefore, "an approach to public policy that assumes that whatever is directed at one age group diminishes another [and] invites policymakers and others to fall into the trap of encouraging intergenerational conflict rather than to seek solutions to problems related to needs that exist across the life course."[8] A different distribution of resources together with a recognition of the malleability of policy, of the continuing possibility of technological progress, and of continuing economic growth could provide a far more optimistic way of thinking about the future of the elderly.

The main focus of the *Common Stake* response, however, was less on those considerations than on the development of a sustained argument in favor of the interdependence of the generations and the adoption of a "life-course perspective." The meaning of generational interdependence is that "at any given point in time, most individuals generally *both give and receive* help. The probability of being more on the receiving than on the giving end changes over the course of life and varies from person to person. The reciprocity of giving and receiving is the bond of *interdependence* that links members of society together."9 The "life-course perspective" points to an important dimension of that interdependence, implying "(1) that quality of life in old age for current and future generations of the elderly is shaped by policies directed at *all* age groups, and (2) that each generation has a clear stake in policies that will shape its well-being at all points throughout the course of life."10 The advantages, the report urges, of these ways of looking at the relationship of the generations in any supposed competition for resources are twofold: they emphasize that people, over the course of their lives, change in their needs and their relationship to different age groups, and that benefits to the generations are reciprocal over time. At any given moment, for example, it is true that the young are transferring massive resources to the elderly in the form of various entitlement programs; and that can seem unfair and unbalanced. But viewed over the course of time, it is a system that means the young will receive similar benefits when they become aged.

This is surely an attractive way of looking at intergenerational equity, one that helpfully defuses the idea that the old and young must necessarily compete for resources. It also has some serious flaws, most notably its failure to confront the historical fact (although there is a passing reference to short-term problems) that the relatively sudden demands made upon resources by the old in recent decades threaten to unbalance any smooth flow of an equitable share of resources from one generation to the next. The argument in *The Ties That Bind* implies that there is no serious problem of allocation of resources to the elderly. Because everyone either is already old or will become old, a social policy of expenditures on the elderly benefits all generations in the long run; that is our "common stake."11 Health-care benefits for the aged also have some immediate value for younger generations. They help relieve the young of burdens of care of the elderly they would otherwise have to bear. Of no less benefit is research on those diseases which particularly affect the elderly. That research also commonly produces health knowledge of pertinence to the young and their diseases as well as bringing the promise of relief, when they are old, from diseases they would otherwise be forced to expect. The young are thus reassured about their own future to a greater extent.

That is, up to a point, plausible enough as a way of unfolding the "life-course perspective," certainly helping to "clarify the reciprocity of giving and receiving that exists between individuals and generations over time."[12] It also obscures some other important considerations. So far at least as health is concerned, it is a view that could be taken to imply that any amount of health care for the old would be beneficial to society because it would benefit everyone else as well. If this is an implication, it does not follow. Too much of a good thing going to one age group could harm other age groups. How much is enough for the elderly? That is the first question to be answered. We must first and independently decide, in the context of comparison with other social needs, just how high a priority health care for the aged should have in relationship to other social goods. In the absence of such a determination, we could not only skew overall social priorities, but also create a particular imbalance over the next few decades. Precisely because the recent successes of medicine have introduced a radical historical and biological distortion into the older patterns of longevity and chronic illness, there is an uncommonly difficult transition problem. How can we envision the good of all age groups simultaneously in the face of that change? Can we somehow find a new vantage point to ask what the "life course" ought to be?

If the aged as a proportion of the population promised to remain stationary over the next few generations, and *if* there were no great chance of an increase in the average life expectancy of the old or in the burden of chronic illness among them, and *if* the odds were against the introduction of further life-extending technologies— then, in that case, a "life-course perspective" could be put immediately to work. But it cannot now rationally be used without the prior exercise of freshly deciding what we want old age to be, what kind and proportion of resources we ought to devote to old age, and what the long-range implications of our choices for both old and young may be. Precisely because the future of aging, medically and socially, is so open-ended, so subject to some conscious ethical and policy decisions, it would be a mistake to simply leap into the middle of a "life-course perspective." We have to fashion that idea anew, taking into account as a necessary first step some basic judgment about how much and what kind of health care would be right for the elderly in the future. A "life-course perspective" does not obviate the need to determine appropriate health care for the elderly, but logically requires it (together with a similar determination for other age groups) as a first step.

If the arguments I have presented in this book are at all sound, moreover, then our present modernization-of-aging approach is mistaken, and so with it the particular "life-course perspective" it entails. It leads inevitably to an inappropriate level of health care for the elderly by its omission of any consideration of limits and by its denial, in practice, that there is even a problem of fair allocation. By its passivity in the face of constant technological progress and the attendant constant redefinition of what the old need, the modernizing ideology forces upon us a competition among the generations that should not exist. We do have a "common stake," but it is first and foremost a stake in determining what are reasonable demands by the generations. Only then are we likely to have any chance of a smooth flow of resources between the generations over time. It may or may not be the case that we can spend more and more on health care for the elderly without dislocating the economy or doing harm to younger generations. That does not seem likely. But a no less important question is whether that would be a good way to spend our money even if we could afford it. It think not: it does not contribute to the long-run welfare of the society as a whole, and it deludes the aging and near-aging into evading the basic question of the meaning and significance of aging and death.

2• Health and Other Values. Could the time be close at hand when it would be justifiable to scale back across-the-board research on the improvement of health, out of an acknowledgment of the great progress already made and the generally good health of most (though, of course, hardly all) people? The 1987 National Institutes of Health budget of $6.2 billion, a 17-percent increase over 1986, is ample testimony to the high place given health in the United States. If there is an indefinite continuation of the widespread belief that health must be endlessly pursued, and all disease and disability understood to be an unmitigated evil, then it is unlikely that any logical limits will be accepted to health care for the aged. This is a delicate and complex issue even to raise. Health is such a high value, so obviously fundamental to human flourishing, that any suggestion that its pursuit should eventually give way to other values and priorities requires some support. No one wants to be ill, and if sickness, disability, and suffering mark a life, they are evils. Is it, then, even possible to envision, and then implement, a different balance between health and other needs than we now have? Short of a cruel and capricious form of budget-slashing, certain to do harm to the elderly, is some balanced outcome along the lines I have proposed even possible?

In practice, of course, health budgets give way all the time to other needs. Only it is rare for direct trade-offs between health care and, say, agricultural subsidies to be made; they just happen as part of the political struggle. Most often the rationale of allocations ordinarily remains obscure within the policy process. It is simply the net outcome of the pressure of competing political forces and interests, the way our system works. But there seems to be an important exception to that rule. If the needs (or interests) of one sector or another of the economy can be dramatized, and if it can be shown that some crucial part of human welfare is tied in with it, money can usually be found and priorities shifted. Budgets for the aged have had that kind of advantage in recent decades, spurred by the rising number and proportion of the elderly, the pragmatic virtue in assisting them, some patent dire needs, and, one must suppose, a recognition of the "common stake" that all generations have in help to the aged: we will all be there someday. An analogous process was visible with the increase of the defense budget during the Reagan years: the President was able to command a great increase in funds because of ideological shifts, economic incentives, and heightened awareness of supposed national-security threats. Presumably one reason for the decline of federal support for programs aiding children was the failure of the groups working in their behalf (weaker by far, in the first place, than those supporting the elderly and national defense) to mount an equally successful case. In an aging society, moreover, there are fewer children proportionately, and their needs less visible or successfully clamorous for attention.

In achieving a more balanced policy on the allocation of health resources to the elderly, two requirements are fundamental. The first is the necessity for public discussion of the comparative needs of different age groups, and precisely as individual age groups. We know that the young need to survive childhood and enter their adult years healthy enough to realize their individual possibilities and to become contributing members of the society. We know that during those adult years they need sufficiently good health to raise families, to manage their lives, and to run the society for which they, as an age group, bear the heaviest responsibility. But what *exactly* do those general needs now entail? Where are the deficiencies, the avoidable premature deaths, the unmet rehabilitation needs, and so on? With a clearer picture of those needs (and "needs" understood with a sharp eye to the distorting influence of desire and technology), we might then be able to view a broader, more integrated panorama to help us make allocation decisions. An unwillingness to look at needs collectively, precisely as *age-group* needs, means that a focus on meeting individual needs obscures shared problems. The young and the old have individual differences and individual needs. They also, for all those differences, as young and old, share common traits and problems within their age groups. It is that full picture, of the needs of each age group placed side by side as equals in our attention, that should be made manifest and then debated.

The second requirement is then to put that picture within one that is still larger: the place of health among other individual and societal needs. Those include economic security, national defense, environmental protection, education of the young and old, industrial development, culture and the arts, basic scientific understanding and research, and spiritual and psychological development. The enormously exciting and beneficial progress of medicine in recent years has given good health a high place. It has become possible and achievable, something not true for earlier generations. Yet the same paradoxes exist for us as for earlier generations. Good health does not guarantee a good life, or a longer life necessarily a better life. A good life is compatible with some degree of poor health, and a life obsessively dedicated to good health can be neurotically miserable, ever threatened by germs, viruses, banana peels, and cold drafts. That I have lived a longer life than Mozart has not, I notice, enhanced my musical potential; and his early death did not leave us utterly bereft of his compositions.

When poor health was common, and death almost equally possible at any age, the passion for something better was only natural. Yet now, in the developed countries, many of the earlier goals have been accomplished. By investing enormous resources in health, we have made it less of a problem for most people; and yet we still spend large amounts of money to do even better. In the meantime, our school and transportation systems have deteriorated, our parks and recreational facilities have not kept pace with population growth and public usage, basic scientific research (save for biomedicine) has lagged, many of our cities continue to deteriorate, our production and economic strength have declined, and a generation of young people find it more difficult than ever to marry, raise children, and buy a home. Quite apart from whether health care for the elderly is the cause of more difficult economic times for young adults (which I doubt is true in any case), it is still possible to ask whether what we collectively spend on everyone for health is money well spent.

Have we, in short, possibly reached a point of diminishing returns—not for some individuals afflicted with terrible diseases, but for our common well-being, happiness, and prosperity? That is possible. We have well passed that point (save for some of the poor and minority groups) at which poor health is the direct cause of any of our nation's major economic or social problems. The marginal improvement in overall health statistics over the next few decades, at increasingly greater cost, is not at all likely to be a key to the nation's greatness, civil peace, prosperity, or national honor, or even the happiness of daily life. Whether that is true or not, however, is well worth a major national debate. In the aftermath of the great health-care revolution of the past fifty years or so, where are we in finding (or even asking about) the appropriate level of good health compatible with those other goods for which we need the health? If we slowed the pace, tried to divert some of the money to, say, public education, would the loss be great? Which would help our common future as a people more: still better health, or something else? Those are remarkably neglected questions, or questions we all too quickly dismiss by saying we could have it all if we were just more efficient, or raised (or lowered) taxes, or cut down the defense or agriculture budget (or government red tape), or whatnot. They are still questions worth asking, urgently so, and utterly appropriate for dialogue between the young and the old in particular.

3• *Medicare and Care of the Aged.* The mounting campaign for cost containment and changes in the Medicare program, for the limitation of long-term institutionalization of the elderly, for both a stronger family role and greater self-help by the elderly add up to a hazardous and unstable mix. Economic considerations are already driving the engine of change. Their prominence signals a readjustment of forces between the public and private spheres, between the family and the welfare state, and between ideas of political entitlement and personal responsibility that mask the advent of thinly disguised rationing strategies. The drive for cost containment, aiming simply to save money, has already shown itself capable of reducing not high-technology tertiary medical care, but those ancillary health and social services which sustain a decent daily quality of life and health for the elderly. A Medicare recipient can receive expensive lifesaving hospital care, but find it impossible to gain support for decent home care once the initial recovery period has passed. As the burden of chronic illness increases, often as the aftermath of successful acute-care interventions, that combination becomes increasingly destructive, certainly for the patient and often enough also for the family forced to provide care in the absence of any alternative. As Rashi Fein has noted: "It is time . . . to face the fact that by cost control we really mean control of expenditures, to be achieved by defining people out of the health system and by shifting costs among the various payers. But shifting costs is hardly equitable, and cutting back on Medicare, Medicaid, and private insurance is a form of rationing. The fact that access is allocated by an impersonal market and invisible hand may make it more acceptable. It hardly makes it more virtuous."[3]

There is, in that respect, good reason to be wary of proposals to make families more responsible for the care of their elderly members. Family life continues to change, and decisively away from conditions that make it congenial for care of the old. The steady increase in single and divorced women, particularly women forced to care for their own children under less-than-ideal circumstances, is itself reason to be strongly skeptical of the mounting enthusiasm for home care. Already there are widespread reports of stress among female workers who must both hold down a job during the day and then care for old and often sick parents at night. Some 25 percent of women, it is estimated, now have that dual responsibility; and it can take a high toll. Voluntary organizations (church and neighborhood groups, for example) can provide some help and relief, but rarely enough to be decisive. That these demographic and domiciliary changes come at a time when cost-minded changes in Social Security and Medicare are discussed and increasingly enacted makes for a discouraging combination. What Samuel Preston said of care for children might also be said of care for the elderly: "we may be returning responsibilities to families not because they are so strong but because they are so weak."[4]

All of this is happening without any kind of coordinated plan or alternative vision of a good life for the elderly. The cuts are being made the same way the programs were originally put into place: piecemeal and opportunistically, flowing and floating with the political tides. W. Andrew Achenbaum is correct when, after surveying the various proposals to reform the Medicare program, he says "The 'health care crisis' is so acute and complex as to demand a new conceptual framework—one that makes it possible to think clearly about what to do and why to do it."[5] Medicare itself should be considered endangered, not because it is likely to be dropped altogether, but because it could be picked and nibbled at in a debilitating way. Despite its shortcomings, Medicare's universalistic incorporation of the elderly represents a communal expression of solidarity between the generations. It preserves, if in a stunted form, a societal commitment to meeting health-care needs on grounds other than relative economic advantage. Given the recent regressions from the 1970s goal of a minimal level of decent health care for all at an affordable price, the importance of Medicare extends beyond those it serves directly as beneficiaries. To the extent that it moves in the direction of the further privatization of burdens of illness and old age, relying on higher premiums, more onerous cost sharing, even means testing, the prospects for reversing current trends in general health policy will be diminished.[16]

I say that to make clear that the broad lines of my proposal about health care for the elderly should not be construed as a way of further weakening Medicare. In most respects, it should be strengthened. Nothing less than a full-blown national health-insurance program, guaranteeing a minimally adequate level of health care for all, will suffice to do justice to the health needs of the elderly as well as to those of other age groups.[17] I am opposed *only* to the ever-widening scope of Medicare coverage for life-extending technological medicine for the elderly. That is where the line must be drawn, but drawn as part of a full-scale rethinking of the goals of medicine and aging. As Henry J. Aaron, a former Assistant Secretary of the Department of Health, Education and Welfare, has observed: "All developed nations face a profound dilemma—to bear the rapidly increasing costs of providing care to aging populations or, alternatively, to ration care, and in so doing deny some potential benefits to some patients."[18]

Why is Congress willing to pay for acute hospital care, to cater to such technological advances as organ transplants for the elderly, but to resist those forms of support which can make the difference not between life and death, but between a good life and a terrible one? No good answer can be found to that question. Yet the former is the kind of care that should be curbed. A Medicare system that clearly and openly established some limits to the most expensive and most problematic care, and to care that extends life well beyond what a person needs to fulfill the major possibilities of life, would show a sensitivity to the deepest needs of the elderly now missing in the present system. More generally, it makes no sense to improve medical care for the elderly while some 35 million Americans have no health insurance at all. That represents an enormous neglect of other age groups. New goals must be shaped in any case for the elderly. Improved social and economic support for family care, for long-term institutional care when required, for assistance in daily living for those elderly able to live alone, for support of the burdens of chronic illness would be worthy goals. The loss of the possibility of added years in the future would more than be compensated for by a heightened exploration, to use Pindar's phrase, of "the limits of the possible."

4• *The Emerging Struggle: Prolife and Antiageism.* When I first learned to sail, the worst days were those when the wind seemed to blow from all directions, gusting one moment from the southwest and the next from the northwest. Those were the days to get hit by the boom. It is not much different trying to find the direction of the political winds of aging. They are blowing from at least three points on the political compass. There is a powerful budget-driven gust, often with bipartisan support, intent on containing costs and reducing costly entitlement programs. It is nervous about picking on programs benefiting the aged, but correctly perceives them to be one of the great fiscal black holes, capable of consuming an ever-larger portion of tax revenues. There is a no less strong countercurrent coming from the various advocacy groups for the aged. Motivated by a belief both in the continuing problems of the elderly and in the important role to be played by government programs in responding to them, it resists all budget cuts and publicizes the many still-unmet needs of the aging. The third gust comes from a relatively new source on the aging compass, that of a "prolife" (sometimes called a right-to-life) movement which has now extended its mission outward from opposing abortion to resisting efforts to change thinking and policy in the care of the dying, especially the elderly dying.

I will comment here only on the latter two movements. They touch directly upon some of the issues that have been just below the surface of my argument, particularly individualism, on the one hand, and the valuation of life, on the other. While both the aging advocacy and the prolife movements are interested in protecting the elderly, there is an important and ultimately clashing set of differences in their premises. Nonetheless, each in its own way is likely to remain an opponent of any wide-ranging effort to reform the system of health care for the elderly, particularly in the direction I have been suggesting. Since these are both important interest and advocacy groups, their viewpoints require attention.

By its emphasis upon the importance of government programs, voluntary community efforts, and facilitating the independence of the elderly, the aging-advocacy movement reveals its roots in the liberalism that has been the mark of the twentieth-century rights and reform movements. The flavor of those roots is displayed by the authors of *The Common Stake* when they write that "In a complex and interdependent society like ours, individual autonomy and independence remain, as they should, cherished values; to maximize these values, we must seek an appropriate balance between individual, family, and governmental efforts."[19] The purpose of government is to provide basic social and medical security, but the ultimate rationale behind that conviction is the need to promote an equal chance to take advantage of life's opportunities and to facilitate freedom of choice in using those opportunities. With the aged (once, and perhaps still) an oppressed and stigmatized group, both their security and their autonomy are in jeopardy.

The prolife movement comes to the issue of aging from a different direction. It sees the legalization of abortion as the first step in a concerted policy to relieve society of the unwanted and burdensome, whether they be fetuses at one end of the life span or the demented elderly at the other. Its leaders want to protect the elderly from the kind of slippery slope of gross indifference to the sacredness of life represented, they believe, by the abortion movement and the more recently alleged trend to cease treating handicapped newborns. "We face," a prominent prolife writer has said, "a pro-death juggernaut."[20] While they share with the aging-advocacy movement a desire to protect the elderly, they are profoundly suspicious of those aspects of it which would increase the liberty of the elderly or their surrogates to terminate treatment. While they are not necessarily unconcerned about cutbacks in entitlement programs for the elderly (though that is not ordinarily touched upon in their literature), their primary focus is on averting the kind of situation that marked Nazi Germany, the systematic neglect and extermination of the undesirable, burdensome, and costly old.

I do not pretend that my brief characterizations by any means catch the nuances, and internal variations, that mark both those movements. As with other movements, their adherents range over a continuum. I would simply underscore the powerful motive in both cases to serve the old, however different may be their underlying ideologies and histories. Both movements also pose severe obstacles, I believe, to some necessary changes in perspective if the elderly are to be well served in the future.

By its stress upon autonomy and the modernizing spirit of which that concept is a central part, the mainline aging-advocacy movement fuels the constant technological advance and redefinition of human and elderly "need" that would do away with all limits, that stands behind Dr. Butler's "push outward without a sense of limits." By seeing aging and society as infinitely malleable, accepting only those (temporary) restraints which our present scientific ignorance imposes upon us, it implicitly refuses to accept aging and death as acceptable parts of human life. As I noted in Chapter 5, it *says* it accepts death, but its actual agenda is a crusade against all the known causes of death. Moreover, despite its emphasis upon the interdependence of the generations, it has an exceedingly anemic social perspective: it can only ask for more for the elderly as individuals because "more" is the modernizing, individualistic, diverting way to deal with the unsettling finitude of life in the absence of real meaning and significance for aging and death. Its apparent ambition to persuade people to think of the aged no longer (save for the purpose of entitlement programs) as part of an identifiable group of people with some common traits, but only as particular individuals with individual needs intensifies that trend. Age as such will not have any special value. The autonomy sought for the aged will be matched by judgment of them on their individual merits and not on their age.

The prolife movement, in its zeal to protect the elderly, also does them some grave disservices. In its persistent opposition even to "living will" legislation, it is prone, in the name of protecting them, to deny the elderly the right to self-determination. By its suspicion of any effort to empower the elderly to terminate their treatment, to choose death rather than more medical care, it then leaves the elderly at the mercy of an aggressive medicine, defenseless to resist an invasion of their bodies that may do them no good and may and often does in actuality increase their suffering. By its seeming belief that life should be preserved under almost all circumstances, it too ends in slavery to technology. By its logic, it must use whatever means are available to save and extend life. Even if not theoretically, there turn out in practice to be no acceptable grounds to refuse to do so. To concede even a first step, one gathers, is to prepare the way for the direct killing of the old, a kind of domino theory of terminating care.

The prolife perspective does not have any evident communal vision either. By an unrelieved, unmodulated stress upon the individual uniqueness of each person combined with a bias toward the preservation of life that often becomes indistinguishable in practice from vitalism, it seems resistant to any larger social understanding of the aged, the passing of the generations, and death. If it does not in theory urge that old age be transformed, treated as a new frontier, that is what it implies in practice. Though often springing from religious roots, the prolife emphasis on preserving individual life does not bring to bear the richer understandings of the nature of a community or a people that are no less a part of the Jewish and Christian traditions. It is as narrowly individual-centered in its own way as the nonreligious liberalism it opposes, and as utterly bereft of any deep view of what old age could or should be.

| What Are We About?

I HAVE TRIED IN THIS BOOK to pose some questions that I believe we as a society must examine. We must ask whether it is good for the elderly, and those of us who will be old in time, to be held hostage to the present course of an ever-restless drive for the improvement of their, and our, future medical lot. We need to know whether it will be forever good for the human community to pursue as an obsessive goal a never-to-be-finished fight against disease and the ravages of age. We should decide whether it will be good for the bonds between the generations to treat the health "needs" of the elderly as morally identical to those of the young, as if death and decline were the equal enemy of both. Those are not simple questions to address, and not only because they are delicate and controversial, touching as they do on some of our most vital personal interests. We also lack good moral and cultural resources to do so.

The individualism of our society is one obstacle. It is more comfortable by far in worrying about improving the lot of individuals than in coping with intergenerational responsibilities, or in struggling to maintain freedom of and financial support for medical research on aging than asking how that freedom ought wisely to be used. The place of the elderly in a good society is a communal, not only an individual, question. It goes unexplored in a culture that does not easily speak the language of community and mutual responsibility. The demands of our interest-group political life constitute another obstacle. It places a high premium on a single-minded pursuit of the interests of particular groups or causes. That is where the usual political rewards are to be found. It is most at home using the language of individual rights as part of its campaigns, and can rarely afford the luxury of publicly recognizing the competing needs of other groups.[21] Yet the greatest obstacle may be our almost utter inability to find a meaningful place in public discourse for suffering and decline in life. They are recognized only as enemies to be fought: with science, with social programs, and with a supreme optimism that with sufficient energy and imagination they can be overcome. We have created a way of life that can only leave serious questions of limits, finitude, the proper ends of human life, of evil and suffering, in the realm of the private self or of religion; they are thus treated as incorrigibly subjective or merely pietistic.

The confusion at the philosophical level is matched by a newly emergent uncertainty as to how we are to understand aging at the political and social levels. This confusion has seen the emergence of a question thought closed some decades ago: whether welfare and medical programs for the aged should be based on criteria of age or of financial need.[22] The premise of the 1935 Social Security and the 1965 Medicare legislation was a calculated decision in favor of using age, not need, as the standard. Yet financial pressure as well as, ironically, the success of gerontologists in persuading the public that age as such tells us little anymore about a person's needs or capacities have now brought that standard into question. Are the aged, as a group, well off or needy? We get mixed, conflicting answers. There has been a condemnation of any stereotyping of the aged, taken to be a symptom of "ageism." Simultaneously, there have also been urgent pleas for better social and health programs to assist the aged, a group with great needs. "The result," as Douglas W. Nelson has noted, "is that the aging movement in America now encompasses and identifies with a range of programs and policies that individually rest on fundamentally incompatible and inconsistent definitions of what it means to be old and on contradictory conceptions of where old people fit into the larger society."[23]

A culture addicted to both individualism and medical progress, and now afflicted by confusion about the legitimate place and needs of the elderly, brings too many problems upon us too fast. What can it mean to say in such a murky context that the aged are now claiming too much of our resources at the expense of the young? "Too much" by what social norms and moral principles? Why don't the elderly have just as strong a claim to resources to meet their needs as any other group, even if their needs are greater? What can it mean to say that the elderly dying cost too much, as if there existed some ethical perspective of an authoritative kind that could decide what is "too much"? The elderly dying can rarely help it if their deaths are expensive; that is part of what it means to be old and sick. Why should that be held against them? What, finally, can it mean to contend that too much high-technology medicine is developed and deployed to the benefit of the elderly rather than to other age groups? Have we not already succeeded in eliminating most of the great killers of the young and thus radically reduced infant and child mortality rates? When the remaining great killers of human beings are conditions mainly afflicting the elderly, and conditions that will benefit from high-technology (albeit expensive) medicine, why should not biomedicine turn its attention in that direction?

Those are the reasonable and inevitable questions that can be thrown against the perspective I am urging. I readily acknowledge their validity and have tried to respond to them. I am also uncomfortably aware of the possibilities for moral mischief in even raising questions, good ones or not, about what we owe the elderly, how much we should spend on them, and what the proper relations between the old and the young in the need for resources should be. Perhaps some questions are best left unanswered and unasked. They are too wrenching, too volatile, too dangerous, and too intractable for acceptable solutions. We can thus continue on the present course, pretending that we are not doing what we are doing—that is, rationing resources to the elderly. "Evasion, disguise, temporizing, deception are all ways by which artfully chosen allocation methods can avoid the appearance of failing to reconcile values in conflict. . . . Averting our eyes enables us to save some lives even when we will not save all."[24] But as the authors of those words quickly note, a strategy of that kind must eventually fail: "We want suffering to end, but it will not. Honesty permits us to know what is to be accepted, and, accepting, to reclaim our humanity and struggle against indignity."[25]

That kind of honesty should now press us to admit that we cannot continue on the present course of open-ended health care for the elderly. Neither confident assertions about our affluence nor tinkering with entitlement provisions nor cost control will work for more than a few more years. It is time for the pretense that old age can be an infinite and open frontier to end and for the unflagging, but self-deceptive, optimism that we can do anything we want with our economic system to be put aside. We will not serve the good of the elderly with the fiction that only a lack of resources, or better financing mechanisms, or political power stands between them and the limitations of their bodies. We will not serve the good of younger generations by inspiring in them a desire to live to an old age that will simply extend the vitality of youth indefinitely, as if old age were nothing but a sign that medicine has failed in its mission. We will not serve the future of our society if we allow spending on health care for the elderly to endlessly escalate, fueled by a false altruism that thinks anything less is to deny the elderly their dignity or by that pervasive kind of self-serving which urges the young to support such a crusade because they will eventually benefit from it also. We can do better.

I have tried to advance three proposals. The first is that in our hopes and our political strategies, we desist from pursuing without prudent limits medical goals that combine these features: the beneficiaries are primarily the elderly, indefinite life extension is sought, the costs are high, and the population-wide benefits are slight. By contrast, we should seek to advance research and health care that increases not the length of life but the quality of life of the elderly. The second proposal is that those who work in behalf of the old shift their priorities from simply gaining more for the elderly, whatever the "more" is, toward the development of an integrated perspective on a natural life span, one that knows where the boundaries are. Not more life but a better life is an attainable goal, one that will benefit the young and the old. The third proposal is that we try to enter into a pervasive cultural agreement to alter our perception of death as an enemy to be held off at all costs to its being, instead, a condition of life to be accepted, if not for our own sake then for that of others. As it happens, that is hardly a new idea. It has just been forgotten or denied in practice, and it is our common task to see if it can be recovered.

Those three proposals lay the foundation for a fresh approach to health care for the elderly. A medicine that accepted as its appropriate goal helping people to live out a full and natural life span, not simply more life without discernible end, would have a plausible and coherent task. The same could be said of a health policy that worked toward helping each age group prevent or avoid as much illness and disability as possible, that provided adequate care when illness struck regardless of ability to pay, that tried to avert premature death, and that sought to enable everyone to live out a natural life span but no more than that. None of that would be possible or plausible without a more sober understanding of old age, one less bemused by dreams of medical liberation and fantasies of bodily transcendence. We require instead an understanding of the process of aging and death that looks to our obligations to the young and to the future, that sees old age as a source of knowledge and insight of value to other age groups, that recognizes the necessity of limits and the acceptance of decline and death, and that values the old for their age and not their continuing youthful vitality.

In the name of accepting the elderly and repudiating discrimination against them, we have mainly succeeded in pretending that old age can be abolished. In the name of meeting the needs of the elderly, we have let commerce and technology, not an analysis of what old age should mean and signify, shape our attitudes and control our behavior. In the name of medical progress we have carried out a relentless war against death and decline, failing to ask in any probing way if that will give us a better society. The proper question is not whether we are succeeding in giving a longer life to the aged. It is whether we are making old age a decent and honorable time of life. Neither a longer lifetime nor more life-extending technology is the way to that goal.

Appendix

Demographic and Health-Care Projections for the Elderly

SOCIAL AND MEDICAL EXPENDITURES of the proportions now encountered in the care and welfare of the elderly cannot fail to catch one's eye, whether first noticed in the family, trying to pay the bills, or in Congress, noting the rapid increase in costs over the past two decades. But why do we have these problems at all, and what are some likely demographic, economic, and medical trends in the future? Let me glance first at some of the most salient data on the increase in life expectancy, the growing proportion of the aged in society, and the costs in health care that those trends bring with them.

For most of the history of the human race, the average life expectancy barely exceeded the age of 30, beginning to rise only in the industrialized world in the eighteenth and nineteenth centuries. It was by no means the case that earlier societies did not have elderly members; if one survived childhood, the chances of living into one's 60s, 70s, and 80s were not impossible. In the eighteenth century in the United States, some 5 percent made it to the age of 60. Even so, it was not until the twentieth century that genuinely dramatic increases in life expectancy appeared. In 1900 there were 3.1 million people over 65, 4.1 percent of the population. Between 1900 and 1984 the number increased eightfold, to 28.0 million, and the percentage to 11.9 percent. No less strikingly, the older generation itself became older: the 75–84 group (8.6 million) was 11 times as large as the same group in 1900, and the number of those 85 and older (2.7 million) was 21 times as great.[1] Life expectancy at age 65 increased by only 2.4 years between 1900 and 1960, but has now increased by 2.5 years since 1960.

Those over 85 are the fastest-growing age group, and the 24-percent increase in their number experienced since only 1960 is projected to increase another 44 percent by 2040. That group, now 1 percent of the population, should rise to 5 percent by 2050, and from 9 to 24 percent of those 65 and older.[2] Where males born between 1929 and 1931 had a life expectancy of 59.8 years and females 61.1, those born in 1984 can expect 76.0 years of life if male and 78.3 if female. By 2050, it is estimated, white males will have a life expectancy of 79.8 years and white females 83.6 years.[3] The life expectancy could, of course, be much greater; earlier projections were much lower than those actually achieved in the 1980s. If the average annual rate of decrease in age-specific death rates that has occurred since 1968 continues for another 65 years, average life expectancy at birth will be 100.[4]

At the same time that lives have been extended, families have been having fewer children. The result is a shift in the ratio of old to young and in the "dependency" or "support" ratio. In 1985 there were 19 elderly for every 100 people of working age, up from a ratio of 7 older people per 100 in 1900. By 2020, the ratio is expected to rise to 29 per hundred, and to 38 per hundred by 2050.[5] In 1985, for the first time in American history, the number of those over 65 exceeded the number of those under 18. While some aged work and some working-age people are not employed, it is still true that the working-age group must heavily support the aged. The total dependency ratio (the ratio of children and elderly to the working-age population) is not expected to show a dramatic change in the coming decades. But the fact that it is primarily public funds that serve the elderly and private funds the young indicates increased demand for public monies as well as growing pressure on families to provide greater social and nonfinancial forms of support.[6]

How heavy will that pressure be? There are two key issues pertinent to any attempt to answer that question. The first is the likely general health of the elderly in the years and decades ahead. The second is the reliability of the projections of health-care needs and costs. While some have predicted a great improvement in the health of the elderly up until the time of death—a "squaring of the curve" of sickness—most studies indicate that an increase in longevity has been matched by an increase in chronic illness. "Longer Life but Worsening Health?" was a question asked by an important article in 1984, and it was answered with a decisive yes. The "worsening health" includes an increase in the average period of diminished vigor, a larger proportion of old age burdened with chronic illness, and a sharp increase in the need for medical care as the number of those over 85 grows dramatically.[7] That there may be increases in both the number who live lives of good health until just before their death and the number who suffer severe disabilities is possible and likely.[8]

There is, then, no special reason to believe that health trends among the aged will bring about a reduction in health-care needs. They will grow at a striking rate. Between 1980 and 2040, the following increases have been projected for those over 65: a 157-percent increase in physician visits, a 197-percent increase in days of hospital care, a 278-percent increase in the number of nursing-home residents, and a 159-percent increase in personal health expenditures (in constant 1980 dollars). Even more striking, and a reflection of the expected increase in chronic illness among the very old, is the 265-percent increase in physician visits by those 75 and over, the 291-percent increase in days of hospital care, and the 318-percent increase in nursing-home residents for the same age group.[9] It is not simply the needs of the old as a group that will become more pronounced (since there will be many variations among them) but particularly the increase of the very old, who will have much higher expenses than the younger old.[10]

Needs of that kind cannot but lead to higher costs. In 1980, 29 percent of personal health-care expenditures were made in behalf of those 65 and over, some $219.4 billion. By 2040, it is projected that the percentage will have increased to 45 percent and the costs (in 1980 dollars) to $369 billion. In 1960, less than 15 percent of the federal budget went to the elderly; it had grown to 28 percent by

1985. During that same period, the proportion going to health care as distinguished from income maintenance under Social Security grew from 6 to 30 percent.[11] The net result is that health-care costs as a whole for the aged are expected to increase from $50 billion in 1978 to almost $200 billion in 2000 (again, in constant 1980 dollars). The portion of total costs that will be borne by public expenditures is expected to go from $29 billion in 1978 to $114 billion in the year 2000.[12] In 1986, pension and health programs were 9.6 percent of the GNP and 39.4 percent of the federal budget. Those figures are projected to jump by 2040 to 14.5 percent of the GNP and 60.4 percent of the budget, respectively.[13]

Notes

CHAPTER 2

1. *Cf.* S. Jay Olshansky and A. Brian Ault, "The Fourth Stage of the Epidemiological Transition: The Age of Delayed Degenerative Disease," *Milbank Memorial Fund Quarterly* 64:3 (1986), p. 361.

2. *Cf.* Gerald J. Gruman, "Cultural Origins of Present-Day 'Ageism': The Modernization of the Life Cycle," in *Aging and the Elderly: Humanistic Perspectives in Gerontology*, ed. Stuart F. Spicker *et al.* (Atlantic Highlands, NJ: Humanities Press, Inc., 1978), pp. 359–87. It should be noted that when I use the term "modernization" I am not using it to refer to "modernization theory" as employed in economics or development theory. For a discussion of the latter see W. Andrew Achenbaum and Peter N. Stearns, "Old Age and Modernization," *Gerontologist* 18 (1978), pp. 307–12.

3. *Ibid.*, p. 380.

4. *Ibid.*, p. 379. For a contrasting way of dealing with death as part of the way of life of a culture see Victor W. Marshall, "Socialization for Impending Death in a Retirement Village," *American Journal of Sociology* 80 (March 1975), pp. 1124–44.

5. *Ibid.*, p. 378.

6. Robert H. Binstock, "The Aged as Scapegoat," *Gerontologist* 23 (1983) p. 142.

7. Arlie Russell Hochschild, "Disengagement Theory: A Logical, Empirical, and Phenomenological Critique," in *Time, Roles, and Self in Old Age*, ed. Jaber F. Gubrium (New York: Human Sciences Press, 1976), pp. 53–87. See also E. Cumming and W. C. Henry, *Growing Old: The Process of Disengagement* (New York: Basic Books, 1961), and B. Neugarten and R. J. Havighurst, "Disengagement Considered in a Cross National Context" In R. J. Havighurst *et al.* eds., *Adjustment to Retirement: A Cross National Study* (The Netherlands: Von Gorcum and Co., 1969).

8. See David Gutmann, "Alternatives to Disengagement: The Old Men of the Highland Druze," in *Time, Roles, and Self in Old Age*, ed. Jaber F. Gubrium (New York: Human Sciences Press, 1976), pp. 88–108.

9. Ronald Blythe, *The View in Winter* (New York: Harcourt Brace Jovanovich, 1979), p. 18.

✓ 10. The best discussion of the harmful effects of modernization ideas on old age is by Harry R. Moody, "The Meaning of Life and the Meaning of Old Age," in *What Does It Mean to Grow Old*, ed. Thomas R. Cole and Sally Gadow (Durham, NC: Duke University Press, 1986), pp. 11–42.

11. Elizabeth Warren Markson, "Readjustment to Time in Old Age: A Life Cycle Approach," *Psychiatry* 36 (February 1973), pp. 37–48.

12. *Cf.* Gutmann, "Alternatives to Disengagement," pp. 107–8.

13. *Cf.* Markson, "Readjustment to Time," p. 45.

✓ 14. Thomas R. Cole, "Aging and Meaning: Our Culture Provides No Compelling Answers." *Generations* 10 (Winter 1985), pp. 49–52: I strongly recommend the writings of Thomas Cole for an understanding of these matters. See especially Cole and Mary G. Winkler, "Aging in Western Medicine and Iconography: History and the Ages of Man," *Medicial Heritage* (September/October 1985), pp. 335–47; Cole, "Aging, Meaning, and Well-Being: Musings of a Cultural Historian," in *Aging 2000: Our Health Care Destiny*, ed. Charles M. Geitz *et al.* (New York: Springer-Verlag, 1985), pp. 361–70; Cole, "The Ideology of Old Age and Death in American History," *American Quarterly* 31 (Summer 1979), pp. 223–31; Cole, "The Prophecy of Senescence: G. Stanley Hall and the Reconstruction of Old Age in America," *Gerontologist* 24 (1984), pp. 360–66; Cole, " 'Putting Off the Old': Middle-Class Morality, Antebellum Protestantism, and the Origins of Ageism," in *Old Age in a Bureaucratic Society: The Elderly, The Experts, and The State in American History*, ed. David Van Tassel and Peter N. Stearns (New York: Greenwood Press, 1986), pp. 49–65.

15. Cole, " 'Putting Off the Old,' " pp. 61–62.

16. Erik H. Erikson, *Insight and Responsibility: Lectures on the Ethical Implications of Psychoanalytic Insight* (1st ed.; New York: W. W. Norton, 1964), pp. 132–33.

17. Erik H. Erikson, *The Life Cycle Completed: A Review* (New York: W. W. Norton, 1982), p. 61. Many of the same ideas are developed in the context of a series of interviews with elderly people in Erik H. Erikson, Joan M. Erikson, and Helen Q. Kivnick, *Vital Involvement in Old Age* (New York: W. W. Norton, 1986).

18. *Ibid.*, p. 62.

19. *Ibid.*, p. 63; see also Edmund Byrne, "Death and Aging in Technopolis: Toward a Role Definition of Wisdom," *Journal of Value Inquiry* 10 (Fall 1976), pp. 161–75.

20. Erikson, *The Life Cycle Completed: A Review*, p. 67.

21. *Ibid.*, p. 63.

22. *Ibid.*

23. *Cf.* Sidney Callahan and Drew Christiansen, "Ideal Old Age," *Soundings* 57 (Spring 1974), pp 1–16.

24. Eric R. Kingson, Barbara A. Hirshorn, and John M. Cornman, *Ties That Bind: The Interdependence of Generations* (Washington, DC: Seven Locks Press, 1986), pp. 51–68.

25. For a good discussion of family support, see Gunhild O. Hagestad, "The

Aging Society as a Context for Family Life," *Daedalus* 115 (Winter 1986), pp. 119–39.

26. A number of valuable efforts have been made in recent decades to provide intergenerational contacts and opportunities for the old to serve the young. They are helpfully summarized in Ira Mothner, *Children and Elders* (New York: Carnegie Corporation of New York, 1985).

27. Alasdair MacIntyre, *After Virtue: A Study in Moral Theory* (Notre Dame, IN: University of Notre Dame Press, 1981), pp. 190, 203.

28. Edmund Burke, *Reflections on the Revolution in France* (London: Dent, 1910), pp. 93–94.

29. Leon R. Kass, *Toward a More Natural Science: Biology and Human Affairs* (New York: Free Press, 1985), p. 315.

30. Simone de Beauvoir, *The Coming of Age*, Translated by Patrick O'Brien (New York: G. P. Putnam's Sons, 1972), p. 28.

31. Harry R. Moody, "The Meaning of Life and Old Age," p. 21.

32. From "On Moral Duties," *Cicero, The Basic Works of Cicero*, ed. Moses Hadas (New York: Modern Library, 1951), p. 47.

33. *Cf.* Cole, "Aging and Meaning," p. 51.

34. William F. May, "Who Cares for the Elderly?" *Hastings Center Report* 12 (December 1982), p. 36.

35. *Ibid.*

CHAPTER 3

1. Ronald Blythe, *The View in Winter: Reflections on Old Age* (New York: Harcourt Brace Jovanovich, 1979), p. 4.

2. John Demos, "Old Age in Early New England," in *Aging, Death, and the Completion of Being*, ed. David D. Van Tassel (Philadelphia: University of Pennsylvania Press, 1979), pp. 122–23.

3. Kenneth G. Manton, "Changing Concepts of Morbidity and Mortality in the Elderly Population," *Milbank Memorial Fund Quarterly* 60:2 (1982), p. 195.

4. *Morbidity and Mortality Weekly Report.* "Annual Summary 1983: Reported Morbidity and Mortality in the United States," 32 (December 1984), p. 108.

5. For a good discussion of the problems of a "thin theory," see Amy Gutmann, "Communitarian Critics of Liberalism," *Philosophy and Public Affairs* 14 (Summer 1985), pp. 308–22; and John Rawls, "Justice as Fairness: Political Not Metaphysical," *Philosophy and Public Affairs* 14:3 (Summer 1985), pp. 223–51.

6. See Robert A. Burt, "Legal Reform and Aging: Current Issues, Troubling Trends," in *What Does It Mean to Grow Old?: Reflections from the Humanities*, ed. Thomas R. Cole and Sally Gadow (Durham, NC: Duke University Press, 1986), pp. 108–9.

7. Leon R. Kass, *Toward a More Natural Science: Biology and Human Affairs.* (New York: Free Press, 1985), p. 169.

8. *Ibid.*, p. 162.

9. *Ibid.*

10. *Ibid.*, p. 163.

11. *Ibid.*, p. 162.

12. *Ibid.*, p. 172.

13. *Ibid.*, pp. 164–68.

14. *Ibid.*, pp. 173–74.

✓ 15. Frank Reynolds, "Natural Death: A History of Religions Perspective," in *Life Span: Values and Life-Extending Technologies*, ed. Robert M. Veatch (San Francisco: Harper and Row, 1979), pp. 153–54. In an earlier article, I tried to develop the concept of a "natural death." ("On Defining a 'Natural Death,' " *Hastings Center Report* 7 [June 1977], pp. 32–37.) I later came to think that the idea of a "natural death" is beset by too much ambiguity to be useful. I would also note that a number of attempts were made in the 19th century to define a concept of a "natural death" and to use that as a way of making death seem more tolerable. Some of that spirit, no doubt, lingered on in my own thinking. For an account of the 19th-century efforts, see James J. Farrell, *Inventing the American Way of Death, 1830–1920* (Philadelphia: Temple University Press, 1980), pp. 51–66.

✓ 16. Timothy F. Murphy, "A Cure for Aging?" *Journal of Medicine and Philosophy* 11 (August 1986), p. 250. Murphy's paper in general takes up an issue I have not discussed in this book, the idea that aging might be considered a disease. See also Arthur L. Caplan, "The Unnaturalness of Aging," in Arthur L. Caplan, H. Tristram Engelhardt, and James McCartney, *Concepts of Health and Disease* (Reading: Addison-Wesley, 1981), pp. 31–85.

✓ 17. Matilda White Riley and John W. Riley, Jr., "Longevity and Social Structure: The Added Years," *Daedalus* 115 (Winter 1986), pp. 53–54.

18. "Prolongevity" has been defined by Gerald J. Gruman as "the significant extension of the length of life by human action." See his masterly essay on the subject, "A History of Ideas About the Prolongation of Life," *Transactions of the American Philosophical Society* 9 (1966), pp. 191–216. For a more recent and scientifically oriented discussion see Albert Rosenfeld, *Prolongevity II* (New York: Alfred A. Knopf, 1985). The moral issues of life extension are well treated in Robert M. Veatch, ed., *Life Span: Values and Life-Extending Technologies* (New York: Harper and Row, 1979).

19. Hans Jonas, *The Imperative of Responsibility* (Chicago: University of Chicago Press, 1984), p. 19. Bernard Williams has provocatively discussed the problem posed for the self by an unending life in "The Makropulos Case: Reflections on the Tedium of Immortality," Chapter 6 in *Problems of the Self* (New York: Cambridge University Press, 1973), pp. 82–100.

20. Kass, *Toward a More Natural Science*, p. 312.

21. *Ibid.*, p. 314, 316.

✓ 22. Eric J. Cassell, "The Nature of Suffering and the Goals of Medicine," *New England Journal of Medicine* 306 (March 1982), p. 640.

23. *Ibid.*, p. 644.

✓ ₦ 24. Lois M. Verbrugge, "Longer Life but Worsening Health? Trends in Health and Mortality of Middle-Aged and Older Persons," *Milbank Memorial Fund Quarterly* 62:3 (Summer 1984), pp. 475–519. It should be noted that Victor Fuchs has reservations about the supposed connection between increasing longevity and growing chronic illness, in " 'Though Much Is Taken': Reflections on Aging, Health, and Medical Care," *Milbank Memorial Fund Quarterly* 62:2 (Spring 1984), pp. 143–66.

25. Ernest M. Gruenberg, "The Failures of Success," *Milbank Memorial Fund Quarterly* 55:1 (Winter 1977), pp. 3–24.

26. M. Kramer, "The Rising Pandemic of Mental Disorders and Associated Chronic Diseases and Disabilities," *Acta Psychiatrica Scandinavica* [*Suppl*] 62 (1980), pp. 382–96. S. Jay Olshansky and A. Brian Ault have provided suggestive evidence of a "postponement of the ages at which degenerative diseases tend to kill" in "The Fourth Stage of the Epidemiologic Transition: The Aged of Delayed Degenerative Diseases," *Milbank Memorial Fund Quarterly* 64:3 (1986), pp. 355–91.

27. James F. Fries, "The Compression of Morbidity," *Milbank Memorial Fund Quarterly* 61:3 (Summer 1983), pp. 347–419; James F. Fries and L. M. Crapo, *Vitality and Aging* (San Francisco: W. H. Freeman Co., 1981).

28. Edward L. Schneider and Jacob A. Brody, "Aging, Natural Death, and the Compression of Morbidity: Another View," *New England Journal of Medicine* 309 (October 1983), pp. 854–56; George C. Myers and Kenneth G. Manton, "Compression of Mortality: Myth or Reality?" *Gerontologist* 24 (August 1984), pp. 346–53.

29. *Cf.* Sidney Katz *et al.*, "Active Life Expectancy," *New England Journal of Medicine* 309 (November 1983), pp. 1218–24.

30. See Matilda White Riley and Kathleen Bond, "Beyond Ageism: Postponing the Onset of Disability," in *Aging in Society: Selected Reviews of Recent Research*, ed. Matilda White Riley *et al.* (Hillsdale, NJ: Erlbaum Associates, 1983), pp. 243–52; and the comment of James M. Fries in "The Compression of Mortality: Miscellaneous Comments About a Theme," *Gerontologist* 24 (August 1984), p. 359: "If the major resources of medicine, as at present, continue to be expended on 'the flat of the curve,' utilizing heroic technology to combat increasingly inevitable death, then both individual morbidity and national medical costs may continue to increase."

CHAPTER 4

1. *Cf.* Mary Joy Quinn, "Elder Abuse and Neglect Raise New Dilemmas," *Generations* 10 (Winter 1985), pp. 22–25.

2. Statement of James L. Scott, Associate Administrator for Operations, Health Care Financing Administration, before the House Select Committee on Human Services, May 16, 1983.

3. Stephen Crystal, *America's Old Age Crisis* (New York: Basic Books, 1982), p. 40.

4. *Ibid.*, p. 52.

5. Ethel Shanas, "The Family Relations of Old People," *National Forum* 62 (Fall 1982), p. 10. As for the motivation behind the visits of children to their parents, Victor Fuchs cites a study purporting to show "that the number of visits was positively related to the parents' bequeathable wealth" in Victor Fuchs, " 'Though Much Is Taken': Reflections on Aging, Health, and Medical Care," *Milbank Memorial Fund Quarterly* 62:2 (Spring 1984), p. 160.

6. James L. Callahan, Jr., *et al.*, "Responsibilities of Families for Their Severely Disabled Elderly," paper prepared by the Brandeis University Health Policy Consortium, July 1979, p. iii.

7. Crystal, *America's Old Age Crisis*, pp. 56–57.

8. *Cf.*, Mary Jo Bane, "Is the Welfare State Replacing the Family?" *Public*

Interest (Winter 1983), pp. 91–101; Eric R. Kingson, Barbara A. Hirshorn, and John M. Cornman, *Ties That Bind: The Interdependence of Generations* (Washington, DC: Seven Locks Press, 1985), p. 62.

9. Daniel Yankelovich, *New Rules: Searching for Self-Fulfillment in a World Turned Upside Down* (New York: Random House, 1981), p. 104.

10. *Cf.* Pamela Doty, "Family Care of the Elderly: The Role of Public Policy," *Milbank Memorial Fund Quarterly* 64 (1986), pp. 34–75.

11. Crystal, *America's Old Age Crisis*, pp. 52ff.

12. Edward A. Wynne, *Social Security: A Reciprocity System Under Pressure* (Boulder, CO: Westview Press, 1980). Nancy Foner has, however, helpfully described the great variety of actual values and practices concerning the care of the elderly in different cultures: "Old and Frail and Everywhere Unequal," *Hastings Center Report* 15 (April 1985), pp. 27–37; and *Ages in Conflict* (New York: Columbia University Press, 1984).

13. David Hackett Fischer, *Growing Old in America* (New York: Oxford University Press, 1978), p. 97.

14. For some pertinent analyses of the present state statutes, see, for example, Paul R. Ober, "Pennsylvania's Family Responsibility Statute—Corruption of Blood and Denial of Equal Protection," *Dickinson Law Review* 77 (1972), pp. 331–51; Gregory G. Sarno, "Constitutionality of Statutory Provision Requiring Reimbursement of Public by Child for Financial Assistance to Aged Parents," *American Law Reports Annotated* 3rd, 75 (1977), pp. 1159–78; W. Walton Garrett, "Filial Responsibility Laws," *Journal of Family Law* 18 (1979–80), pp. 793–818; James L. Lopes, "Filial Support and Family Solidarity," *Pacific Law Journal* 6 (July 1975), pp. 508–35.

15. *Commentaries on the Laws of England* Vol. 1 (Philadelphia: J. B. Lippincott and Co., 1856), book 1, ch. 16, section 1, cited in Jeffrey Blustein, *Parents and Children: The Ethics of the Family* (New York: Oxford University Press, 1982), p. 181. It is worth noting that the People's Republic of China apparently persists in upholding stringent filial obligations. The Constitution of 1982 states that "children who have come of age have the duty to support and assist their parents"; and the Marriage Law of 1980 says that "When children fail to perform the duty of supporting their parents, parents who have lost the ability to work or have difficulties in providing for themselves have the right to demand that their children pay for their support." Cited in Alice and Sidney Goldstein, "The Challenge of an Aging Population in the People's Republic of China." Paper presented at annual meeting of Population Association of America, May 3–5, 1984, Minneapolis, MN.

16. See especially W. Walton Garrett, "Filial Responsibility Laws," pp. 793–96.

17. Martin R. Levy and Sara W. Gross, "Constitutional Implications of Support Laws," *University of Richmond Law Review* 13 (1979), p. 523.

18. *Ibid.*, p. 524.

19. *Ibid.*, p. 525.

20. *Ibid.*

21. *Ibid.*, p. 526.

22. *Ibid.*, p. 527.

23. *Ibid.*, pp. 527–28.

24. Jane English, "What Do Grown Children Owe Their Parents?" in Onora O'Neill and William Ruddick, ed., *Having Children: Philosophical and Legal Reflec-*

tions on Parenthood (New York: Oxford University Press, 1979), p. 351; see also ✓
Christina Hoff Sommers, "Filial Morality," *Journal of Philosophy* 33 (August 1986),
pp. 439–56.

25. *Ibid.*, p. 353.

26. Blustein, *The Ethics of the Family*, p. 177.

27. Joel Feinberg, "Duties, Rights, and Claims," *American Philosophical Quarterly* 3 (1966), p. 139; cited in Blustein, *ibid.*, p. 176.

28. Ferdinand Schoeman, "Rights of Children, Rights of Parents, and the Moral ✓
Basis of the Family," *Ethics* 91 (October 1980), p. 8.

29. *Cf.* Robert E. Goodin, *Protecting the Vulnerable: A Reanalysis of Our Social* ✓
Responsibilities. (Chicago: University of Chicago Press, 1985).

30. For further helpful discussions on the general topic, see Andrew Joseph
Christiansen, "Autonomy and Dependence in Old Age," Yale University doctoral
dissertation, 1982; Abraham Monk, "Family Supports in Old Age," *Social Work*
(November 1979), pp. 533–38; Wilma T. Donahue, "What About Our
Responsibility to the Abandoned Elderly?" *Gerontologist* 18 (1978), pp. 102–11;
Wayne C. Seelbach, "Correlates of Aged Parents' Filial Responsibility
Expectations and Realizations," *Family Coordinator* (October 1978), pp. 341–50;
Stanley J. Brody *et al.*, "The Family Caring Unit: A Major Consideration in the
Long-Term Support System," *Gerontologist* 18 (1978), pp. 16–20; Elizabeth S.
Johnson and Barbara J. Bursk, "The Relationship Between the Elderly and Their
Adult Children," *Gerontologist* 17 (1977), pp. 90–96; Alvin Schorr, ". . . Thy
Father and Thy Mother: A Second Look at Filial Responsibility and Family
Policy," U.S. Department of Health and Human Services, SSA Publication No.
13-11953 (Washington DC: Government Printing Office, July 1980); W. Andrew
Achenbaum, *Old Age in the New Land* (Baltimore: Johns Hopkins Press, 1978), pp.
75–80; Joanne P. Ackford, "Reducing Medicaid Expenditures Through Family
Responsibility: Critique of a Recent Proposal," *American Journal of Law and
Medicine* 5 (Spring 1979), pp. 59–79; "Relative Responsibility," *Nursing Home Law
Letter* (February 1982), pp. 1–8.

31. W. Andrew Achenbaum, *Shades of Gray: Old Age, American Values, and Fed-* ✓
eral Policies Since 1920. (Boston: Little, Brown and Company, 1983), pp. 158ff. A
somewhat different version of the ideas presented in this section will appear in a
forthcoming issue of *The Archives of Physical Medicine and Rehabilitation*.

32. *Cf.* Elaine M. Brody, "Parent Care as a Normative Family Stress," *Geron-* ✓
tologist 25 (1985), pp. 19–29; Gunhild O. Hagestad, "The Aging Society as a
Context for Family Life," *Daedalus* 115 (Winter 1986), pp. 119–39.

33. *Cf.* Nancy R. Hooyman and Wendy Lustbader, *Taking Care: Supporting Older* ✓
People and Their Families. (New York: The Free Press, 1986); Betty H. Landsberger,
Long-Term Care for the Elderly: A Comparative View of Layers of Care. (New York: St.
Martin's Press, 1985).

34. Elaine M. Brody, " 'Women in the Middle' and Family Help to Older
People," *Gerontologist* 21 (1985), pp. 471–80; *Caregivers of the Frail Elderly: A National Profile*, study by National Center for Health Services Research (NCHSR),
U.S. Department of Health and Human Services (USDHHS), 1986.

35. *Cf.* William H. Jarrett, "Caregiving Within Kinship Systems: Is Affection
Really Necessary?" *The Gerontologist* 25 (1985), pp. 5–10.

36. Michael Ignatieff, *The Needs of Strangers: An Essay on Privacy, Solidarity, and the Politics of Being Human* (New York: Viking Press, 1984), pp. 52–53.

37. Judith Jarvis Thompson seems to speak for many in moral philosophy when she writes, "surely we do not have any 'special responsibility' for a person unless we have assumed it, explicitly or implicitly," in "A Defense of Abortion," *Philosophy and Public Affairs* 1:1 (1971), p. 65. See also J. D. Urmson, "Saints and Heroes," *Essays in Moral Philosophy*, ed. A. I. Melden, (Seattle: University of Washington Press, 1958), pp. 198–216; and Millard Shoemaker, *Supererogation* (Edmonton, Alberta: St. Stephen's College, 1977).

38. *Cf.* Gene Outka, *Agape: An Ethical Analysis*. (New Haven: Yale University Press, 1972).

39. Judith Tormey, "Exploitation, Oppression and Self-Sacrifice," in *Women and Philosophy*, ed. Carol C. Gould and Marx W. Wartofsky (New York: G. P. Putnam's Sons, 1976), p. 219.

40. *Ibid.*, p. 220.

41. Stephen Post, unpublished paper, personal communication.

42. *Ibid.*

43. June Axinn and Mark J. Stern, "Age and Dependency: Children and the Aged in American Social Policy," *Milbank Memorial Fund Quarterly* 63:4 (Fall 1985), p. 652; see also Jill S. Quadagno, "From Poor Laws to Pensions: The Evolution of Economic Support for the Aged in England and America," *Milbank Memorial Fund Quarterly* 62:3 (Summer 1984), pp. 417–66.

44. Fischer, *Growing Old in America*, p. 224.

45. W. Andrew Achenbaum, "The Meaning of Risks, Rights, and Responsibilities in Aging America," in *What Does It Mean to Grow Old?: Reflections from the Humanities*, ed. Thomas R. Cole and Sally Gadow (Durham, NC: Duke University Press, 1986), pp. 63–98.

46. *Ibid.*, p. 78.

47. Robert Stevens and Rosemary Stevens, *Welfare Medicine in America* (New York: The Free Press, 1974), p. 7.

48. Eric R. Kingson, Barbara A. Hirshorn, and Linda K. Harootyan, *The Common Stake: The Interdependence of Generations* (Washington, DC: The Gerontological Society of America, 1986).

49. Douglas W. Nelson, "Alternative Images of Old Age as the Bases for Policy," in *Age or Need?: Public Policies for Older People*, ed. Bernice L. Neugarten (Beverly Hills: Sage Publications, 1982), p. 157.

50. Achenbaum, "Risks, Rights, and Responsibilities," p. 80.

51. Quoted by Irving Kristol in a review of Ben Wattenberg's *The Good News Is the Bad News Is Wrong* (New York: Simon and Schuster, 1984), in *The New Republic* (October 29, 1984), p. 37.

52. Norman Daniels, "Family Responsibility Initiatives and Justice Between Age Groups." *Law, Medicine and Health Care* (September 1985), pp. 154–55.

53. This theme is eloquently analyzed in Eric R. Kingson, Barbara A. Hirshorn, and John Cornman, *Ties That Bind: The Interdependence of Generations* (Washington, D.C.: Seven Locks Press, 1986).

54. Louis Lowy, "The Older Generation: What Is Due, What Is Owed?" *Social Casework* 64 (June 1983), pp. 374*ff.*

CHAPTER 5

1. Carroll L. Estes, "Social Security: The Social Construction of a Crisis," *Milbank Memorial Fund Quarterly* 61:3 (Summer 1983), pp. 445–61.

2. *A Profile of Older Americans: 1985*, American Association of Retired Persons (AARP), Washington, DC; Dorothy P. Rice, "The Medical Care System: Past Trends and Future Projections," *New York Medical Quarterly* 6 (1986), pp. 39–70.

3. See Daniel R. Waldo and Helen C. Lazenby, "Demographic Characteristics and Health Care Use and Expenditures by the Aged in the United States: 1977–1984," *Health Care Financing Review* 6 (Fall 1984), pp. 1–29.

4. Rice, "Past Trends and Future Projections," p. 61.

5. *Ibid.*, p. 46.

6. Karen Davis, "Aging and the Health-Care System: Economic and Structural Issues," *Daedalus* 115 (Winter 1986), pp. 234–35. Dr. Davis does, however, in another place say that "Extended life expectancy and improved health of the elderly will bring with it a cost—one that is clearly affordable to a growing and prosperous society": in Karen Davis and Diane Rowland, *Medicare Policy* (Baltimore: Johns Hopkins Press, 1983), p. 33. She does not explain why an "increase from about $83 billion in 1981 to almost $200 billion in 2000, in constant 1980 dollars" (*ibid.*) is "clearly affordable," much less whether it would be wise.

7. Robert H. Binstock, "The Aged as a Scapegoat," *Gerontologist* 23 (1983), pp. 136–43; "The Oldest Old: A Fresh Perspective or Compassionate Ageism Revisited?" *Milbank Memorial Fund Quarterly* 63:1 (Spring 1985), pp. 420–51; Bernice L. Neugarten and Dail A. Neugarten, "Age in the Aging Society," *Daedalus* 115 (Winter 1986), pp. 31–49.

8. Samuel H. Preston, "Children and the Elderly: Divergent Paths for America's Dependents," *Demography* 21 (November 1984), p. 435.

9. *Cf.* Binstock, "Scapegoat."

10. Thomas Halper, "The Double-Edged Sword: Paternalism as a Policy in the Problems of Aging," *Milbank Memorial Fund Quarterly* 58:3 (1980), p. 486; Fernando Torres-Gil and Jon Pynoos, "Long-Term Care Policy and Interest Group Struggles," *Gerontologist* 26:5 (1986), pp. 488–95.

11. Roger W. Evans, "Health Care Technology and the Inevitability of Resource Allocation and Rationing Decisions," *Journal of the American Medical Association* 249 (April 1983), pp. 2047–53, 2208–19.

12. *Ibid.*, p. 2052.

13. Henry J. Aaron and William B. Schwartz, *The Painful Prescription: Rationing Hospital Care.* (Washington, DC: The Brookings Institution, 1984).

14. The comparative figures are: United Kingdom, 6.2 percent; Canada, 8.5 percent; Denmark, 6.6 percent; France, 9.3 percent; Japan, 6.7 percent; Netherlands, 8.8 percent; Sweden, 9.6 percent. John K. Iglehart, "Canada's Health Care System," *New England Journal of Medicine* 315:3 (July 1986), p. 205.

15. Binstock, "Scapegoat," p. 139; see also Noralou P. Roos *et al.*, "Aging and the Demand for Health Services: Which Aged and Whose Demand?" *Gerontologist* 24:1 (1984), pp. 31–36.

16. Marcia Angell, "Cost Containment and the Physician," *Journal of the American Medical Association* 254 (September 1985), p. 1204. Erdman B. Palmore has argued that a trend toward better health among the elderly should reduce their

health-care costs: "Trends in the Health of the Aged," *Gerontologist* 26:3 (1986), pp. 298–302. That seems to me optimistic and not supported by other trends.

17. Robert H. Brook and Kathleen N. Lohr, "Will We Need to Ration Effective Health Care?" in press, *Issues in Science and Technology* (National Academy of Sciences).

18. Arthur L. Caplan, "A New Dilemma: Quality, Ethics and Expansive Medical Technologies," *New York Medical Quarterly* 6 (1986), p. 23.

19. John Wennberg and Alan Gittlesohn, "Variations in Medical Care Among Small Areas," *Scientific American* 246:4 (April 1982), pp. 120–34.

20. Uwe E. Reinhardt, "Battle Over Medical Costs Isn't Over," *Wall Street Journal*, October 22, 1986, p. 16. See also William B. Schwartz, "The Inevitable Failure of Current Cost-Containment Strategies," *Journal of the American Medical Association* 257 (January 1987), pp. 220–24.

21. P.L. 99-509, Sixth Omnibus Reconciliation Act (SOBRA), Conference Report, October 18, 1986.

22. B. Torrey, "Guns Versus Canes: The Fiscal Implications of an Aging Population," *American Economic Review* 72 (1982), p. 309ff.

23. Angell, "Cost Containment," p. 1207.

24. *Cf.* Norman Daniels, "Why Saying No to Patients in the United States Is So Hard: Cost Containment, Justice, and Provider Autonomy," *New England Journal of Medicine* 314 (May 1986), pp. 1380–83.

25. This argument is developed at length in Eric R. Kingson, Barbara A. Hirshorn, and John M. Cornman, *Ties That Bind: The Interdependence of Generations* (Washington, DC: Seven Locks Press, 1986).

26. *Ibid.*, p. 26.

27. Victor R. Fuchs, "Though Much Is Taken: Reflections on Aging, Health, and Medical Care," *Milbank Memorial Fund Quarterly* 62:1 (Spring 1984), pp. 464–65.

28. J. Lubitz and R. Prihoda, "Uses and Costs of Medicare Services in the Last Two Years of Life," *Health Care Financing Review* 5 (Spring 1984), pp. 117–31.

29. See Ronald Bayer, Daniel Callahan, *et al.*, "The Care of the Terminally Ill: Morality and Economics," *New England Journal of Medicine* 309 (December 1983), pp. 1490–94.

30. A. S. Detsky *et al.*, "Prognosis, Survival, and the Expenditure of Hospital Resources for Patients in an Intensive-Care Unit," *New England Journal of Medicine* 305 (1981), p. 668.

31. Lubitz and Prihoda, "Costs of Medicare Services," p. 122.

32. Anne A. Scitovsky, " 'The High Cost of Dying': What Do the Data Show?" *Milbank Memorial Fund Quarterly* 62:4 (Fall 1984), pp. 606–7.

33. *Ibid.*

34. Anne A. Scitovsky and Alexander M. Capron, "Medical Care at the End of Life: The Interaction of Economics and Ethics," *Annual Review of Public Health* 7 (1986), p. 71; and Anne A. Scitovsky, "Medical Care Expenditures in the Last Twelve Months of Life" (unpublished paper, March 1986).

35. Norman Daniels, *Just Health Care*. (Cambridge: Cambridge University Press, 1985), pp. 104–5.

36. Norman Daniels, "Family Responsibility Initiatives and Justice Between Age Groups," *Law, Medicine and Health Care* (September 1985), p. 156; *cf.* Phillip

G. Clark, "The Social Allocation of Health Care Resources: Ethical Dilemmas in Age-Group Competition," *Gerontologist* 25 (April 1985), pp. 119–25; and B. J. Diggs, "The Ethics of Providing for the Economic Well-Being of the Aged," in Bernice L. Neugarten and Robert J. Havighurst, ed., *Social Policy, Social Ethics, and the Aging Society* (Washington, D.C.: GPO, 038-000-0029-6).

37. Daniels, *Just Health Care*, p. 106.

38. This general definition is drawn from *Guidelines on the Termination of Life-Sustaining Treatment and the Case of Dying*, Susan Wolf, Daniel Callahan, Bruce Jennings, Cynthia B. Cohen, eds. (Briarcliff Manor, N.Y.: The Hastings Center, 1987), Introduction.

39. One of the first articles to explore the idea of an age basis for allocation was Harry R. Moody's "Is It Right to Allocate Health Care Resources on Grounds of Age?" in Elsie L. Bandman and Bertram Bandman, *Bioethics and Human Rights* (Boston: Little, Brown, 1978), pp. 197–201.

40. For a good general discussion of age as an allocation principle, see Leslie Pickering Francis, "Poverty, Age Discrimination, and Health Care," in George R. Lucas, Jr., ed., *Poverty, Justice, and the Law* (Lanham, MD: University Press of America, 1986), pp. 117–29.

41. Bernice L. Neugarten, ed., *Age or Need?: Public Policies for Older People.* (Beverly Hills: Sage Publications, 1982); see Douglas W. Nelson, "Alternative Images of Old Age as the Bases for Policy," in *Age or Need*, ed. Neugarten.

42. Neugarten and Neugarten, "Age in the Aging Society," p. 47.

43. Jerome L. Avorn, "Benefit and Cost Analysis in Geriatric Care: Turning Age Discrimination into Health Policy," *New England Journal of Medicine* 310 (May 1984), pp. 1294–1301.

44. Carole Haber has written well on this problem in *Beyond Sixty-Five: The Dilemma of Old Age in America's Past* (New York: Cambridge University Press, 1983), especially pp. 125–29.

45. "Life-Sustaining Technologies and the Elderly: Ethical Issues," Chapter 4 of U.S. Congress, Office of Technology Assessment, Biological Applications Program, *Life-Sustaining Technologies and the Elderly* (Washington, D.C.: OTA, July 1987).

46. James F. Childress, "Ensuring Care, Respect, and Fairness for the Elderly," *Hastings Center Report* 14 (October 1984), p. 29.

47. Mark Siegler, "Should Age be a Criterion in Health Care?" *Hastings Center Report* 14 (October 1984), p. 25.

48. Jerome L. Avorn, "Medicine, Health, and the Geriatric Transformation," *Daedalus* 115 (Winter 1986), p. 213.

49. Summarized in *The Washington Post* (July 30, 1986), p. A6, and forthcoming in *Health Care Financing Review* in 1987. See also Geroge E. Thibault *et al.*, "Medical Intensive Care: Indications, Interventions, and Outcomes," *New England Journal of Medicine* 302 (April 1980), pp. 938–42; and Edward W. Campion *et al.*, "Medical Intensive Care for the Elderly: A Study of Current Use, Costs, and Outcomes," *Journal of the American Medical Association* 246 (November 1981), pp. 2052–56.

50. Richard B. Freeman, "Treatment of Chronic Renal Failure: An Update," *New England Journal of Medicine* 312 (February 1985), pp. 577–79; see also Roger

Evans *et al.*, "The Quality of Life of Patients with End-Stage Renal Disease," *New England Journal of Medicine* 312 (February 1985), pp. 553–59.

51. Arthur L. Caplan, "Organ Transplants: The Costs of Success," *Hastings Center Report* 13 (December 1983), pp. 23–32.

52. Alonzo L. Plough, *Borrowed Time: Artificial Organs and the Politics of Extending Lives* (Philadelphia: Temple University Press, 1986). For an example of "age creep" in the use of technology see "Cardiac Surgery in High Risk Octogenarians," *Journal of the American Medical Association* 256 (November 1986), p. 2669. In 1986, a liver transplant was carried out on a 76-year-old patient. "As Liver Transplants Grow More Common, Ethical Issues Multiply, " *Wall Street Journal* 208 (October 14, 1986), p. 1. See also Karen Davis and Diane Rowland, *Medicare Policy*, p. 26.

53. Louis P. Garrison, Jr., and Gail R. Wilensky, "Cost Containment and Technology," *Health Affairs* 5:2 (Summer 1986), p. 50.

54. Kenneth L. Minaker and John Rowe, "Health and Disease Among the Oldest Old: A Clincial Perspective," *Milbank Memorial Fund Quarterly* 63:2 (Spring 1985), p. 343.

55. For an analysis of the problem of encouraging appropriate technologies while controlling costs, see *Technology and Aging in America* (Washington, DC: Congressional Office of Technology Assessment, OTA-BA-264, June 1985); and Garrison and Wilensky, "Cost Containment and Technology."

56. *Aging America: Trends and Projections*, 1985–86 Edition; John L. Palmer and Stephanie G. Gould, "The Economic Consequences of an Aging Society," *Daedalus* 115 (Winter 1986), pp. 295–323.

57. Older Women's League, *Report on the Status of Midlife and Older Women in America* (1986).

58. Rice, "Past Trends and Future Projections," p. 55.

59. See Karen Davis and Diane Rowland, *Medicare Policy* (Baltimore: Johns Hopkins Press, 1986).

60. Janet D. Perloff *et al.*, "Premature Death in the United States: Years of Life Lost and Health Priorities," *Journal of Public Health Policy* (June 1984), pp. 167–84. See also John W. Rowe, "Health Care of the Elderly," *New England Journal of Medicine* 312 (March 1985), pp. 827–834.

61. I am particularly indebted for that information to Janet F. Haas, M.D. and other colleagues who were part of a Hastings Center project on ethical issues in rehabilitation medicine 1985–87.

62. Louise B. Russell, *Is Prevention Better than Cure?* (Washington, DC: The Brookings Institution, 1986).

63. *Ibid.*, p. 111.

64. *Ibid.*

65. For a good discussion of coercion and prevention, see Childress, "Ensuring Care, Respect, and Fairness for the Elderly"; Daniel I. Wikler, "Persuasion and Coercion for Health: Ethical Issues in Government Efforts to Change Life Styles," *Milbank Memorial Fund Quarterly* 56:3 (Summer 1978), pp. 303–38; and a special section, "Voluntary Health Risks," in the *Hastings Center Report*, 11:5 (October 1981), pp. 26–44.

66. *Aging America*, p. 98. See also Anne R. Somers, "Long-Term Care for the Elderly and Disabled," *New England Journal of Medicine* 307 (July 1982), pp. 221–26;

and Terrie Wettle, "Long Term Care: A Taxonomy of Issues," *Generations* 10 (Winter 1985), pp. 30–34.

67. Dorothy P. Rice and Jacob J. Feldman, "Living Longer in the United States: Demographic Changes and Health Needs of the Elderly," *Milbank Memorial Fund Quarterly* 61:3 (Summer 1983), pp. 362–96.

68. Frances H. Miller and Graham A. H. Miller, "*The Painful Prescription*: A Procrustean Perspective?" *New England Journal of Medicine* 314 (May 1986), p. 1385; *cf.* Aaron and Schwartz, *The Painful Prescription*. I should emphasize that the British health-care system seems in considerable trouble at present, in great part because of the financial difficulties of the country and diminishing resources allocated to the National Health Service. More people are opting to buy additional private care, and resources for the elderly are in particular in danger. See Keith Andrews, "Demographic Changes and Resources for the Elderly," *British Medical Journal* 290 (April 1985), pp. 1023–24.

69. Iglehart, "Canada's Health Care System," p. 205.

70. Daniels, "Family Responsibility Initiatives," p. 57.

71. *Cf.* W. Andrew Achenbaum, *Shades of Gray: Old Age, American Values, and Federal Policies Since 1920* (Boston: Little, Brown, 1983), p. 125; Paul T. Menzel, *Medical Costs, Moral Choices: A Philosophy of Health Care Economics in America* (New Haven: Yale University Press, 1983), pp. 193*ff.*

72. I profited in thinking about this issue from reading the manuscript of Norman Daniels' new book *Am I My Parents' Keeper?* particularly his notion of "the prudential lifespan account."

CHAPTER 6

1. The Gallup Poll (March 14, 1985).

2. U.S. Congress Office of Technology Assessment, Biological Applications Program, *Life- Sustaining Technologies and the Elderly* (Washington, D.C.: OTA, July 1987), pp. 1–22*ff.*

3. I have adapted this description from a similar one developed by Jerome L. Avorn, "Medicine, Health, and the Geriatric Transformation," *Daedalus* 115 (Winter 1986), pp. 215–17.

4. This quotation as well as the summaries and further quotations are from OTA, pp. I-39–45.

5. Malcolm Cowley, *The View from Eighty* (New York: Penguin Books, 1982), p. 5. That line was quoted in G. C. Prado's remarkably interesting book *Rethinking How We Age* (Westport, CT: Greenwood Press, 1986) which analyzes psychological and social age, as distinguished from biological age.

6. Mark Siegler, "Should Age Be a Criterion in Health Care?" *Hastings Center Report* 14 (October 1984), p. 27.

7. James F. Childress, "Ensuring Care, Respect, and Fairness for the Elderly," *Hastings Center Report* 14 (October 1984), p. 29.

8. For a full discussion of the rights of competent patients, see President's Commission for the Study of Ethical Problems in Medicine and Biomedical and Behavioral Research, *Deciding to Forgo Life-Sustaining Treatment: Ethical, Medical, and Legal Issues in Treatment Decisions.* (Washington, D.C.: Government Printing

Office, 1983). See also Steven A. Levenson, "Ethical Considerations in Critical and Terminal Illness in the Elderly," *Journal of the American Geriatrics Society* 29:12 (December 1981), pp. 563–67.

9. This theme is developed more fully in Susan Wolf, Daniel Callahan, Bruce Jennings, Cynthia Cohen, eds., *Guidelines on the Termination of Life-Sustaining Treatment and the Care of the Dying.* (Briarcliff Manor, N.Y.: The Hastings Center, 1987).

10. A thorough discussion can be found in Jay Katz, *The Silent World of Doctor and Patient* (New York: Free Press, 1984).

11. Steven Neu and Carl M. Kjellstrand, "Stopping Long-Term Dialysis: An Empirical Study of Withdrawal of Life-Supporting Treatment," *New England Journal of Medicine* 314 (January 1986), pp. 14–20.

12. R. Reiss, "Moral and Ethical Issues in Geriatric Surgery," *Journal of Medical Ethics* 6 (1980), pp. 71–77.

13. The most thorough and balanced analysis of the concept of "quality of life" is that of Edward W. Keyserlingk, *Sanctity of Life or Quality of Life* (Montreal: Law Reform Commission of Canada, 1979); see also Richard McCormick, "The Quality of Life, the Sanctity of Life," *Hastings Center Report* (February 1978), pp. 30–36.

14. John D. Arras nicely develops these distinctions in "Quality of Life in Neonatal Ethics" (unpublished paper presented at Hastings Center, May 7, 1986). The difference between patient and physician judgment of "quality of life" is interestingly discussed in T. Jolene Starr et al., "Quality of Life and Resuscitation Decisions in Elderly Patients," *Journal of General Internal Medicine* 1 (November/December 1986), pp. 373–79. See also David C. Thomasma, "Ethical Judgments of Quality of Life in the Care of the Aged," *Journal of the American Geriatrics Society* 32:7 (July 1984), pp. 525–27.

15. See Cynthia B. Cohen, " 'Quality of Life' and the Analogy with the Nazis," *Journal of Medicine and Philosophy* 8 (1983), pp. 113–35.

16. See Robert J. Lifton's chapter (Chapter 2) " 'Euthanasia': Direct Medical Killing," in *The Nazi Doctors* (New York: Basic Books, 1986), pp. 45– 56, for a good historical analysis of the origin and nature of Nazi attitudes toward killing the sick and handicapped.

17. James Rachels, in *The End of Life: Euthanasia and Morality* (Oxford: Oxford University Press, 1986), p. 5, makes use of this phrase in a helpful way (though I do not support his analysis of euthanasia).

18. I have adapted this classification system from Sidney H. Wanzer et al., "The Physician's Responsibility Toward Hopelessly Ill Patients," *New England Journal of Medicine* 310 (April 1984), pp. 955–59.

19. David Hilfiker, "Allowing the Debilitated to Die: Facing Our Ethical Choices," *New England Journal of Medicine* 308 (March 1983), p. 718.

20. B. Jennett and F. Plum, "Persistent Vegetative State After Brain Damage: A Syndrome in Search of a Name," *Lancet* 1 (1972), pp. 734–37. *Cf.* Ronald E. Cranford, "Termination of Treatment in the Persistent Vegetative State," *Seminars in Neurology* 4:1 (March 1984), pp. 36–44.

21. See especially Joanne Lynn and James F. Childress, "Must Patients Always Be Given Food and Water?" in *By No Extraordinary Means: The Choice to Forgo Life-Sustaining Food and Water*, ed. Joanne Lynn (Bloomington: Indiana University

Press, 1986); see also Daniel Callahan, "Public Policy and The Cessation of Nutrition," in Lynn, *By No Extraordinary Means*, pp. 61–66, and "On Feeding the Dying," *Hastings Center Report* 13 (October 1983), p. 22. An earlier version of material in this section appeared in "Feeding The Elderly Dying," *Generations* 10 (Winter 1985), pp. 15–17.

22. For some criticisms of proposals to withhold hydration and nutrition see Gilbert Meilander, "On Removing Food and Water: Against the Stream," *Hastings Center Report* (December 1984), pp. 11–13; Mark Siegler and Alan J. Weisbard, "Against the Emerging Stream: Should Fluids and Nutritional Support Be Discontinued?" *Archives of Internal Medicine* 145 (January 1985), pp. 129–31; John R. Connery, "The Ethical Standards for Withholding/Withdrawing Nutrition and Hydration," *Issues in Law and Medicine* 2:2 (September 1986), pp. 87–97; Robert Barry, "Facing Hard Cases: The Ethics of Assisted Feeding," in the same issue, pp. 99–115.

23. Paul Ramsey, *The Patient as a Person* (New Haven: Yale University Press, 1970), esp. Chapter 3.

24. James F. Childress, "When Is It Morally Justifiable to Discontinue Medical Nutrition and Hydration?" in Lynn, *By No Extraordinary Means*, pp. 74ff.

25. See Mary Howell, "Caretakers' Views on Responsibilities for the Care of the Demented Elderly," *Journal of the American Geriatrics Society* 32 (September 1984), pp. 657–60, for a sensitive discussion of the relationship between caregivers and the demented; and for another sensitive analysis, see Christine K. Cassel, "Ethical Issues in Dementia," *Seminars in Neurology* 4:1 (March 1984), pp. 92–97. See also Ronald Dworkin, "Philosophical Issues in Senile Dementia," Contract prepared for the Office of Technology Assessment, U.S. Congress, August 1986 (draft); George S. Robertson, "Dealing with the Brain-Damaged Elderly," *Journal of Medical Ethics* 8 (1982), pp. 173–79; and Ralph Goldman, "Ethical Confrontations in the Incapacitated Elderly," *Journal of the American Geriatric Society* 29:6 (June 1981), pp. 241–45.

26. *Cf.* Rachels, *The End of Life*, p. 180. See also Diane E. Meier and Christine K. Cassel, "Euthanasia in Old Age," *Journal of the American Geriatric Society* 31:5 (May 1983), pp. 294–98; and Arthur J. Dyck, "Ethical Aspects of Care for the Dying Incompetent," *Journal of the American Geriatric Society* 32:9 (September 1984), pp. 661–64.

27. Doris Portwood, *Common Sense Suicide: The Final Right* (Los Angeles: The Hemlock Society, 1978), p. 10.

28. Derek Humphry and Ann Wickett, *The Right to Die: Understanding Euthanasia* (New York: Harper and Row, 1986), pp. 206ff. and *passim*. See also Margaret P. Battin, "Age Rationing and the Just Distribution of Health Care: Is There a Duty to Die?" *Ethics* 97 (January 1987), pp. 317–340.

29. Robert S. Morison, "Biological Eschatology," in *Visions of Apocalypse: End or Rebirth?* ed. Saul Friedlander (New York: Holmes and Meier, 1986), p. 147.

30. See *Hemlock Quarterly* Issue 24 (July 1986) for a summary of such polls.

31. Humphry and Wicket, *The Right to Die*, p. 133.

32. *Ibid.*

33. Herbert Hendin, *Suicide in America* (New York: W. W. Norton, 1982), especially Chapter 3, "Suicide Among Older People," pp. 59–82. See also Seymour

Perlin, ed., *A Handbook for the Study of Suicide* (New York: Oxford University Press, 1975). See also Shirley Bromberg and Christine K. Cassel, "Suicide in the Elderly," *Journal of the American Geriatrics Society* 31 (November 1983), pp. 698–703.

CHAPTER 7

1. Robert N. Butler, *Why Survive?: Being Old In America*. (New York: Harper and Row, 1975), pp. 421–22.

2. *Ibid.*, p. 12.

3. *Ibid.*, pp. 6–11.

4. Harold A. Richman and Matthew W. Stagner, "Children: Treasured Resource or Forgotten Minority," in Alan Pifer and Lydia Bronte, *Our Aging Society: Paradox and Promise* (New York: W. W. Norton, 1986), p. 169.

5. Samuel H. Preston, "Children and the Elderly: Divergent Paths for America's Dependents," *Demography* 21 (November 1984), pp. 491–52.

6. Americans for Generational Equity (AGE), Case Statement (May 1986). The issue of "intergenerational equity" is also explored in a thoughtful and provocative way in Phillip Longman, *Born to Pay: The New Politics of Aging* (Boston: Houghton-Mifflin, forthcoming, 1988).

7. Eric R. Kingson, Barbara A. Hirshorn, and John Cornman, *Ties That Bind: The Interdependence of Generations* (Washington, DC: Seven Locks Press, 1986), and Kingson, Hirshorn, and Linda K. Harootyan, *The Common Stake* (Washington, DC: American Gerontological Society, 1986).

8. Kingson, Hirshorn, and Cornman, *Ties That Bind*, p. 154.

9. *Ibid.*, p. 24.

10. *Ibid.*, p. 26.

11. *Ibid.*

12. *Ibid.*, p. 26. I should emphasize that my reservations about the life-course perspective are directed only at its use as a way of defusing possible competition between the generations. *Cf.* Matilda White Riley, ed. *Aging from Birth to Death* (Boulder, CO: Westview Press, 1979).

13. Rashi Fein, *Medicial Care, Medical Costs* (Cambridge: Harvard University Press, 1986), p. 215.

14. Preston, "Children and the Elderly," p. 452.

15. Two valuable studies of Medicare reform—though marked by undue optimism—are Karen Davis and Diane Rowland, *Medicare Policy: New Directions for Health and Long-Term Care* (Baltimore: Johns Hopkins Press, 1986); and Harvard Medicare Project, *Medicare Coming of Age* (Cambridge: Kennedy School of Government, 1986).

16. W. Andrew Achenbaum, *Social Security: Visions and Revisions* (New York: Cambridge University Press, 1986), p. 178.

17. The case for a comprehensive health-care system is nicely developed by Achenbaum in his book *Social Security: Visions and Revisions*. See also the valuable report of the President's Commission, *Securing Access to Health Care* (Washington, DC: Government Printing Office, 1983).

18. Henry J. Aaron, "When Is a Burden Not a Burden? The Elderly in America," *The Brookings Review* (Summer 1986), p. 24.

19. Kingson, Hirshorn, and Cornman, *Ties That Bind*, pp. 160–61.

20. David Andrusko, "Who Is Next?" *New York State Right to Life Newsletter* (August/September 1986), p. 2.

21. See Robert H. Binstock, "The Aged as a Scapegoat," *Gerontologist* 23:2 (1983), p. 142.

22. Bernice L. Neugarten, ed., *Age or Need? Public Policies for Older People* (Beverly Hills: Sage Publications, 1982).

23. Douglas W. Nelson, "Alternative Images of Old Age as the Bases for Policy," in *Age or Need? Public Policies for Older People*, pp. 138–39.

24. Guido Calabresi and Philip Bobbitt, *Tragic Choices* (New York: W. W. Norton, 1978), p. 26.

25. *Ibid.*

APPENDIX: DEMOGRAPHIC AND HEALTH-CARE DATA

1. *A Profile of Older Americans: 1985* (brochure), American Association of Retired Persons (AARP), Washington, DC

2. A Profile of Older Americans: 1985; *Milbank Memorial Fund Quarterly* 63:2 (Spring 1985), special issue, "The Oldest Old."

3. Jacob S. Siegel and Cynthia M. Taeuber, "Demographic Perspectives on ✓ the Long-Lived Society," *Daedalus* 115 (Winter 1986), p. 94.

4. *Ibid.*, p. 98.

5. U.S. Senate Special Committee on Aging, *Aging America: Trends and Projections*, (Washington, DC: U.S. Department of Health and Human Services, 1985), pp. 20–21.

6. See Henry J. Aaron, "When Is a Burden Not a Burden? The Elderly in America," *The Brookings Review* (Summer 1986), pp. 17–24, for a helpful discussion of dependency ratios.

7. Dorothy P. Rice, "The Medical Care System: Past Trends and Future Projections," *New York Medical Quarterly* 6:1 (1986), pp. 39–70; Lois M. Verbrugge, "Longer Life but Worsening Health?: Trends in Health and Mortality of Middle-Aged and Older Persons," *Milbank Memorial Fund Quarterly* 62:3 (Summer 1984), pp. 475–519. See Victor R. Fuchs, " 'Though Much Is Taken': Reflections on Aging, Health, and Medical Care," *Milbank Memorial Fund Quarterly* 62:2 (Spring 1984), p. 146, for a somewhat different viewpoint.

8. Rice, "Past Trends and Future Projections," p. 46.

9. *Ibid.*, p. 63.

10. John L. Palmer and Stephanie G. Gould, "The Economic Consequences of an Aging Society," *Daedalus* 115 (Winter 1986), p. 313.

11. *Aging America*, p. 122.

12. Karen Davis, "Aging and the Health Care System: Economic and Structural Issues," *Daedalus* 115 (Winter 1986), p. 236.

13. *Aging America*, p. 126.

Index